# Summer Body Recipes

My Best Collection of Low Carb, Healthy & Fresh Unprocessed

Food Recipes

By Paula C. Henderson

Paula C. Henderson

**Copyright Page**

# Contents

*"Crave A Healthy Life"*

~ Paula C. Henderson

# OTHER PUBLICATIONS

**From Healthy Food Advocate and Author Paula C. Henderson**

Paula's books are available in kindle and paperback versions. You can see all of her titles on her author's page on Amazon:
**www.amazon.com/author/paulachenderson**

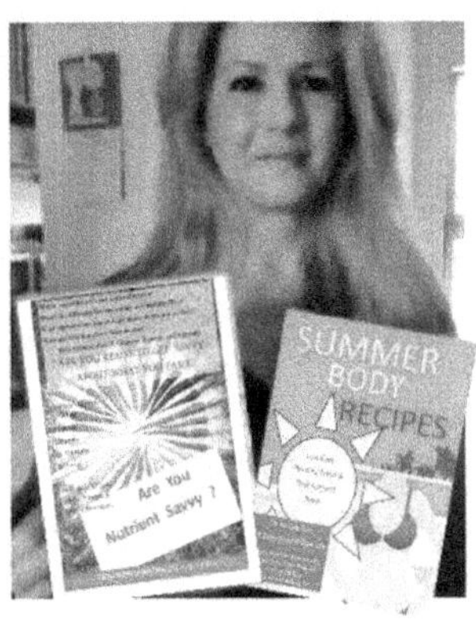

Paula C. Henderson makes her home in Las Vegas, Nevada. Paula grew up in Illinois and then moved to Ohio where, as a single mother, raised her daughter.

Becoming a certified weight loss counselor started an interest in healthy food choices and a healthy lifestyle that continues today.

Taking care of one's self is even more important when facing daily challenges. Through the years Paula has continued her education as a Nutritionist and health care advocate.

- The recipes and information in this book are not so much about being thin and attractive as they are about being healthy. The healthiest you is the best you.
- There is no reason to go hungry if you are trying to lose excess weight. Changing what you are eating and increasing your activity level every single day is my best advice. So, if you feel hungry, eat. Just choose naturally low carb, unprocessed, fresh foods when you do.
- Gluten free does not mean low carb. Check your labels if you are eating gluten free packaged foods, and compare them. For example: A gluten free tortilla may have 24 carbs per tortilla whereas a low carb whole wheat tortilla may only have 7 carbs per tortilla. If you are eating gluten free due to health issues restrict the amount of gluten free packaged foods if you are trying to lose weight.
- Substitutions are okay! Try fried or baked Portobello mushrooms in place of bacon (toss the sliced portabellas in oil, salt and pepper before cooking). Bacon does not have carbs of course but if you are watching your fat or sodium intake you might try the mushroom.
- Almond Milk (original unsweetened) is a great sub for dairy milk or soy milk. I did a side by side taste test of unflavored Almond Milk that was sweetened and the unsweetened original Almond Milk. I did not taste a difference. No reason to consume extra sugars and carbs unnecessarily.
- Cheese does not have carbs so feel free to add cheese to any recipe and know that you are in keeping with a low carb diet. I have excluded cheese from any of the recipes since I wanted these recipes to be dairy free. Dairy is a known inflammatory and many have sensitivities or allergies to dairy.
- There are several recipes you may want to have a bit more heat. You can add crushed red pepper or jalapeños as they do not have carbohydrates. I have excluded them because they are nightshades, known to trigger inflammation.
- All sugars, even healthy sugars from fruits, are carbs. Berries have the lowest carb count of all the fruit. Either avoid fruit all

together, or restrict you diet to just low carb fruits and even then, be sure to be mindful of your portion sizes.

- Many of us have a dulled palate after years of eating overly processed foods. This is why many of you feel vegetables taste bland. In fact, most do not taste bland but you will need to cleanse your palate in order to experience this fact. Challenge yourself to go 45 consecutive days without processed foods. This will cleanse your palate and you will be surprised how much better fresh, healthy, unprocessed foods taste. Like squash and broccoli among others. Overly processed foods generally are higher in carbs. Another reason to avoid them for the next 45 days.

- When a recipe calls for eggs pay attention to the size of egg if referenced. Whole eggs and egg whites will add liquid to a recipe and so in this case, size does really matter!

- Are you eating dairy free? Most dairy products contain casein, but not all. Since casein is a protein, it is found in dairy products that have a higher protein content, such as milk, yogurt, kefir, cheese and ice cream. Dairy products that contain barely any protein, such as real butter and cream, only have traces of casein. Many find they can tolerate real butter on occasion just fine, and so, you will find some recipes in this book using real butter. You can always omit the butter though and use your favorite butter alternative or healthy oil.

- I suggest reading the label of everything in your kitchen. Everything. Take note of the ingredients list if there is one. Are there more than 3 ingredients? If the answer is yes, you may want to omit that product from your diet. Take note of the carb count, sugars, calories, serving size in relation to the amount of product as a whole. Pay attention to fat content and sodium amounts.

# Ingredients List

What ingredients are used in this cookbook? Following is a list of all the ingredients used in the recipes included here, in this cookbook. I have grouped the ingredients by the department of your grocery store where you would find each one. There are certainly other foods that can be included in the healthy low carb groups. I have included a Carb Chart (next chapter) which includes more foods then just those ingredients needed to make the recipes included in this cookbook as many of the recipes here are open to substituting fresh healthy ingredients you may have on hand.

Notice the natural amounts of sodium in our healthy foods. Sodium is a necessary nutrient for the body to function properly, but we get the necessary amounts from our fresh unprocessed foods. No need to add unnecessary amounts as with packaged, processed foods or at the table.

## PRODUCE DEPARTMENT:

Asparagus - per cup: 5 carbs, 2.8g fiber, 3g protein, 3 mg sodium

Avocado - per medium avocado: 17 carbs, 13.5g fiber, 4g protein, 14mg sodium

Broccoli - per cup: 6 carbs, 2 g fiber, 3 g protein, 30mg sodium

Brussels sprouts – per cup: 8 carbs, 3.3g fiber, 3g protein, 22mg sodium

Cabbage (variety) – per cup: 5 carbs, 2g fiber, 2g protein, 16mg sodium

Cauliflower – per cup: 5 carbs, 2.5g fiber, 2g protein, 30mg sodium

Carrots – per cup: 12 carbs, 4g fiber, 1g protein, 88mg sodium

Celery – per cup: 1 carb, 1g fiber, .5g protein, 32mg sodium

Cucumber  -  per 1 cup: 3 carbs, 1g fiber, 1g protein, 3mg sodium

Cilantro – per cup: 0.5 carbs, 0.5g fiber, 0.33g protein, 7mg sodium

Fennel – per ½ cup: 3 carbs, 2g fiber, 1g protein, 80mg sodium

Garlic – per clove: 1 carb, 0.1g fiber, 0.19g protein, 1mg sodium

Green beans – per cup: 8 carbs, 4g fiber, 2g protein, 7mg sodium

Kale – per 1 cup: 7 carbs, 2g fiber, 2g protein, 29mg sodium

Lettuce (variety) – per 1 cup Romaine: 1 carb, 0.5g fiber, 1g protein, 10mg sodium

Lemons and limes – per 1 fruit: 5 carbs, 2g fiber, 1g protein, 1mg sodium

Mushrooms (variety) – per 1 cup: 4 carbs, 2g fiber, 2g protein, 5mg sodium

Onions – per one cup: 16 carbs, 3g fiber, 2g protein, 5mg sodium

Parsley – per 1 cup: 4 carbs, 2g fiber, 2g protein, 34mg sodium

Radishes – per 1 cup: 4 carbs, 2g fiber, 1g protein, 45mg sodium

Scallions – per 1 cup: 7 carbs, 3g fiber, 2g protein, 16mg sodium

Snow peas – per 1 cup: 5 carbs, 2g fiber, 2g protein, 3mg sodium

Spaghetti squash – per 1 cup: 10 carbs, 2g fiber, 1g protein, 330mg sodium

Spinach – per 1 cup: 1 carb, 1g fiber, 1g protein, 24mg sodium

Swiss chard – per 1 cup: 1carb, 1g fiber, 1g protein, 77mg sodium

Zucchini – per 1 cup: 4 carbs, 2g fiber, 2g protein, 12mg sodium

Nutritional data from fatsecret


**REFRIGERATED SECTION:**

Almond Milk (Unflavored Original) – per 1 cup: 1 carb, 1g fiber, 1g protein, 125mg sodium.
   *refer to the label of your milk choice*

Eggs – per 1 egg: 0 carb, 0 fiber, 6g protein, 70mg sodium

*There are some people who eat dairy free that can tolerate Real Butter. If you cannot, simply replace it with your favorite healthy oil or butter alternative.*

Real Unsalted Butter – per 1 Tablespoon: 0 carbs, 0 fiber, 0 protein, 0 sodium

***BEVERAGES:***
***Ingredients for recipes:*** *White Wine or Vermouth*
*Sparkling water (unflavored and add fresh lemon or lime)*
*Tea*
*Coffee*
*Water*

## FROZEN FOODS:

Whole frozen brussels sprouts
Whole frozen okra – per 1 cup: 7 carbs, 3g fiber, 2g protein, 8mg sodium

## BAKING AISLE:

Almond flour – per ¼ cup: 6 carbs, 3g fiber, 6g protein, 0 sodium
Baking Powder – per 1 teaspoon: 1 carb, 0 fiber, 0 protein, 488mg sodium
Brown sugar – per 1 teaspoon: 3 carbs, 0 fiber, 0 protein, 1mg sodium
Coconut flour – per 2 tablespoons: 8 carbs, 6g fiber, 2g protein, 10mg sodium
Cornstarch – per 1 tablespoon: 7 carbs, 0 fiber, 0 protein, 0 sodium
Flaxseed meal – per 2 tablespoons: 4 carbs, 4g fiber, 3g protein, 5mg sodium
Gluten Free Bisquick – per 2 tablespoons: 12 carbs, 0.5g fiber, 1g protein, 136mg sodium
Nuts (variety) – per ¼ cup unsalted: 6 carbs, 2g fiber, 6g protein, 0 sodium
Sunflower Seeds – per ¼ cup unsalted: 6 carbs, 3g fiber, 7g protein, 0 sodium
White Sugar – per 1 teaspoon: 4 carbs, 0 fiber, 0 protein, 0 sodium
Xanthan Gum – per 1 tablespoon: 7 carbs, 7g fiber, 0 protein, 10mg sodium

*Nutritional data taken from actual packaging. Brands may vary. Check your package labels.*

## SPICES AND SEASONINGS:

Bay leaf
Celery seed
Cumin
Garlic powder
Ginger
Italian seasoning
Lemon pepper
Onion powder
Oregano
Pepper
Rosemary
Sage
Salt
Thyme

## MEAT AND SEAFOOD:

Bacon – per 2 slices: 0 carbs, 0 fiber, 4g protein, 160mg sodium
Beef shank bone-in – per 1 pound: 0 carbs, 0 fiber, 93g protein, 272mg sodium
Chicken breasts – per boneless/skinless piece: 0 carb, 0 fiber, 27g protein, 77mg protein
Ground hamburger (preferably grass fed) – per 4 ounces: 0 carbs, 0 fiber, 21g protein, 75mg sodium
Ground pork (Styrofoam, not the tubes) – per 4 ounces: 0 carbs, 0 fiber, 16g protein, 730mg sodium
Ground turkey (Styrofoam, not the tubes) – 0 carbs, 0 fiber, 23g protein, 91mg sodium
Hen
Pork chops
Pork tenderloin
Salmon – per fillet: 0 carb, 0 fiber, 23g protein, 240mg sodium
Shrimp – per one medium shrimp: 0 carb, 0 fiber, 1g protein, 9mg sodium

## CANNED, JARRED, OR BOXED

Apple cider vinegar (raw unfiltered with the mother)
Artichokes
Balsamic vinegar (not balsamic vinegar dressing)
Capers
Chicken broth
Coconut aminos (or soy sauce if you consume soy)
Coconut oil
Dijon mustard
Dill pickle relish
Horseradish
Kraut

*For nutritional data on packaged foods, check your packaging as brands may vary.*

Mayonnaise (homemade or your favorite healthy brand)
Oil (preferably olive oil, avocado oil, coconut oil or walnut oil)
Olives
Salmon (boneless skinless) (could substitute tuna)
Sesame seed oil
Red wine vinegar
Rice wine vinegar
Stevia

# Carbohydrate Chart

The recommendation, according to the Mayo Clinic, for daily carb consumption, is 225-325 carbs per day in order to maintain your weight if on a standard recommended 2000 calorie per day diet.

*To be consuming what is overall viewed as a low carb diet, one must keep daily carb consumption to 100 or less carbs per day.*

**Zero to 4 carbs per serving: If you choose from this list as the bulk of your diet you can significantly cut down your daily carb intake. Some but not all of these foods are used in the recipes that follow.**

All meats and seafood
Apricot (fresh)
Asparagus
Avocado
Avocado oil
Broccoli
Broth (make homemade broth. If you buy broth, check the label)
Cabbage
Cauliflower
Celery
Club soda
Coconut
Coconut oil
Coffee (unsweetened, no dairy added)
Cucumbers
Dried spices overall (not seasoning packets)
Eggs
Fennel
Fish oil
Garlic
Green beans

Grass fed Real Unsalted Butter
Hearts of Palm
Horseradish
Kraut
Lard
Leafy greens like kale, lettuce (all), bok choy, spinach, turnip greens, parsley, cilantro, etc
Lemons and limes
Mayo (check the label though)
Mushrooms (all)
Mustard (for the most part. Check your ingredient labels)
Non-gluten vinegars (not malt vinegar for example)
Nuts
Okra
Olives
Olive oil
Onions
Pumpkin (if limited to ½ cup servings)
Radish
Raspberries (the lowest of the berries)
Seeds
Snow peas
Spaghetti squash
Sparkling water
Stevia
Tea
Tequila
Walnut oil
Water
Yellow squash
Zucchini

# A Word about Fruit

We all love our fruit. Especially in the summer. However, even healthy sugars are sugars and all sugars are carbs. Having said that, if you want to include some fresh cold fruit in your diet this summer be sure to consider these findings:

**Cantaloupe** is even considered low carb when limited to one slice (about 9 carbs) especially when compared to a banana which has approximately 25 carbs. The average **apple** has about 15 carbs, so if you eat an **apple** choose one that is especially small.

A peach is another good choice at about 7 carbs for a small fresh peach. Avoid canned peaches and avoid peaches that are especially large.

An **orange** has about 15 carbs

**Blackberries**: per one cup has about 12 carbs

**Strawberries**: per one cup has about 12 carbs

**Watermelon**, per one cup servings: 12 carbs

Choose a **tangerine** (instead of an orange) and get just 9 carbs

**Peaches** average about 9 carbs per medium size fruit.

One average size **plum** has 7 carbs

One **Apricot** has just 4 carbs!

**Honey**, an alternative, whole foods sweetener has 17 carbs per tablespoon. So, if you use it, try keeping it to ½ teaspoon per day, or 1 tablespoon once per week, if any at all.

# Suggested Meals and Substitutions:

Grilling is almost always a good way to go for a healthy way to prepare your foods.

Many of these recipes are flexible in that if it calls for Swiss chard or spinach, you could easily replace with kale if you have kale on hand and prefer it. Kale is a wonderfully healthy food with zero carbs. The same goes for meats and seafood's. I have a pork chop recipe, but round steak would work nicely too!

*A favorite here is simply steak and zucchini on the grill. Prepare your favorite steaks and along with that include grilled zucchini: Slice fresh zucchini in half lengthwise. Rub with oil, salt and pepper and grill until tender and a nice golden brown in color.*

A healthy guacamole can be a nice substitute for mayonnaise.

Cucumbers quite literally liquefy when blended in a blender with just a tad of water and you can turn that into a very healthy salad dressing! Just add a bit of oil, vinegar and seasonings. I have a few salad dressing recipes included in the book and one or two begin with and/or include a cucumber as the base. You can thicken it up using an avocado or a can of drained, pureed artichokes.

If you are preparing a recipe and not sure about one of the ingredients you are supposed to add next and how it will taste; Say you are making a sauce and you have most of it in the skillet and then it calls for a spice you aren't sure you will like. Remove a bit of the sauce into a small bowl. Add a touch of the spice you are not sure of and give it a taste.

## What should your plate look like?

Vegetables should be *at least* half your plate. Meat, seafood or your protein should be just ¼ of your plate and the last quarter of your plate should be a fresh element. Your fresh element could be sliced cucumber, salad, salsa verde, slaw, or parts of a fresh vegetable tray.

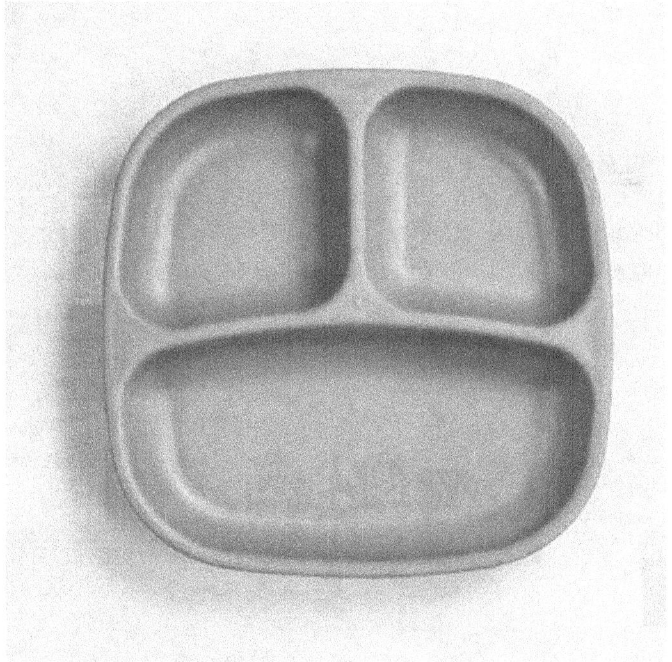

Summertime!

May, June, July, and August

Four months. 122 Days. About 16 weeks.

Beginning weight: May 1st _________________
Weigh in May 31st           _________________

Weigh in June 30th          _________________

Weigh in July 31st          _________________

Weigh in August 30          _________________

You might also want to track your symptoms from obesity, thyroid, arthritis and other common health issues stemming from overeating, high carb diets, gluten, dairy, nightshades and soy. A fresh healthy diet is naturally low in carbs! Don't forget that sugar is a carb.

SYMPTOMS

After 2 months:

After 4 months:

# 18  BREAKFAST RECIPES

Before presenting you with some low carb healthy breakfast ideas and recipes let me first state that I firmly believe there are no harden rules on what constitutes a breakfast food. I regularly eat warm pureed carrots in the winter months and sometimes, especially in the summer, I have fresh cucumbers for breakfast. So loosen up on approved ingredients for your breakfast. Eat what you like that is healthy, fresh and low carb.

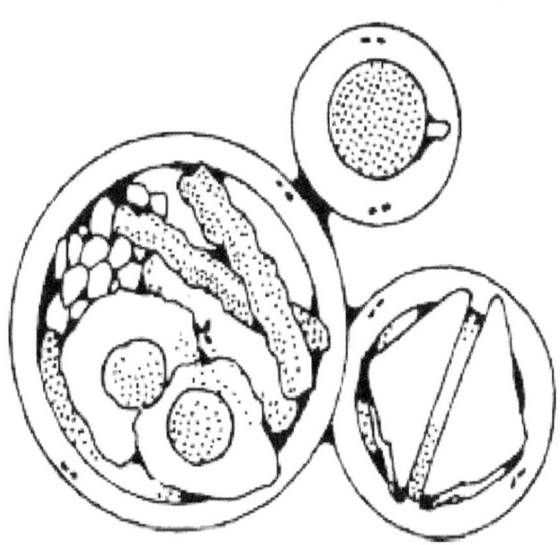

# Recipe 01: Avocado Toast

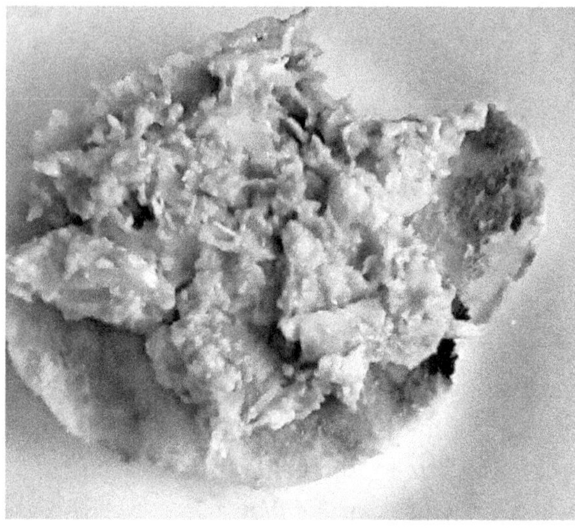

Ripe avocado either slices or mashed; whichever you prefer

Your toast can be your choice too! You can use the Drop biscuit recipe 07; slicing the biscuit in half and toasting it nice and crispy before adding your avo. Slice a pre-made drop biscuit, put in your toaster oven until crispy toasty brown.

You can use your favorite store bought low carb bread.

I will sometimes use the Pizza Crust Recipe 54. Especially when making a pizza crust over the weekend and I may make an extra one to use during the week.

Below is another quick microwave toast method you might like to try. The texture is that of cornmeal or say a triscuit cracker. This "English muffin" recipe below is what I used in the picture above.

**INGREDIENTS**:

- 3 T. Almond flour
- 1 t. coconut flour
- 1 T. melted solid oil (Real Unsalted Butter, Ghee, or Refined Coconut Oil)
- 1 large egg (not an extra-large. If all you have is extra-large: whisk the egg in a small bowl and only use most, but not all! About ¾'s of the egg)
- A pinch of salt
- ½ t. baking powder

Best prepared in a 4 inch diameter microwave safe ramekin or container with a near flat bottom.

1.  In your container of choice combine all the ingredients. Be sure your oil is melted. Do not use oil. Use something you must melt. Stir quickly together making sure all of the ingredients are completely blended.
2.  Allow this to sit for at least 2 full minutes until appears "set".
3.  Microwave for exactly 90 seconds. Should be released from the sides of the dish.
4.  Let cool for about 2 minutes. Using a butter knife, loosen the edges and turn the bread over onto a plate. Cut in half and then toast. An oven, toaster oven, or skillet is recommended but I have used the toaster; in fact, the picture above was toasted in a traditional toaster.

This toast will seem quite dry if you just bite into it. But, it does go well with butter, oil, or even a runny egg on top as it has all of those wonderful nooks and crannies.

According to the USDA National Nutrient Database, one serving (one-fifth of an avocado, approximately 40 grams) contains:

64 calories, 3.4 carbs, less than a gram of sugar, almost 3 grams of fiber

Avocados are a great source of vitamins C, E, K, B-6, riboflavin, niacin, folate, pantothenic acid, magnesium, and potassium, lutein, beta-carotene, and omega-3 fatty acids.

# Recipe 02: Biscuits and Gravy

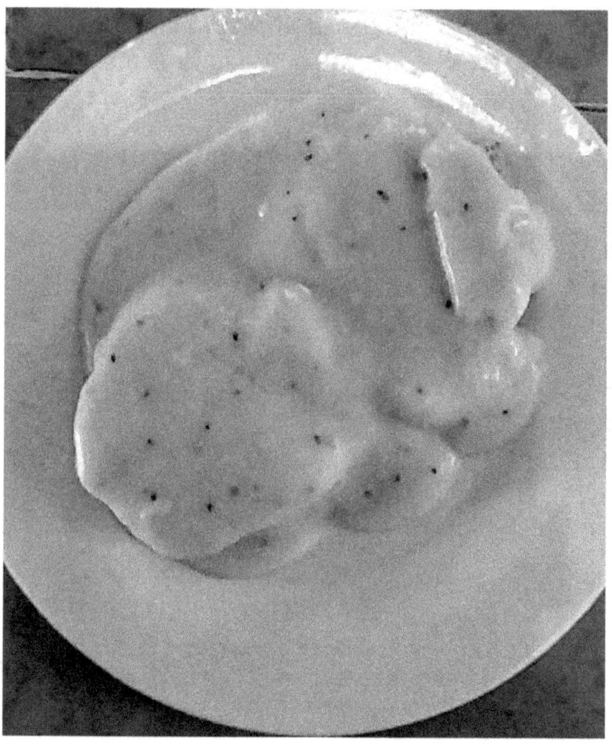

A hearty breakfast for big appetites.

Use the biscuit recipe from Recipe 07: Drop Biscuits
And Recipe 18: Sausage Gravy (the gravy in this picture depicts one without the sausage. I used real unsalted butter in place of the fat rendered from meat). You will use the fat rendered from your ground pork or bacon if you include a breakfast meat in the gravy.

I am using Almond Flour in place of a traditional wheat or white flour. Almond flour has 6 carbs per ¼ cup whereas all purpose flour has 23 carbs per ¼ cup.

I also used unflavored original Almond Milk to make the gravy. My favorite non-dairy milk go-to!

# Recipe 03: Breakfast Pizza

Pizza Crust Recipe 54
And your choice of topping!
Some suggestions:
Cooked Bacon, sausage or ham
Eggs: scrambled, boiled, or fried
Mushrooms
Avocado

I like to use the Breakfast Salad Recipe 04 to place on top of my pizza crust. No need to return to the oven. I don't really consider a "sauce" for my breakfast pizza as I simply use it as I would a piece of toast or English muffin and do not normally put a sauce on my breakfast sandwiches.

However you could use the sausage gravy, Recipe 18 in the Breakfast chapter and then top with scrambled eggs or a fried egg like a breakfast bowl. Another idea would be to spread cauliflower hash browns recipe 06 in breakfasts, and then top that with a runny fried egg or poached egg.

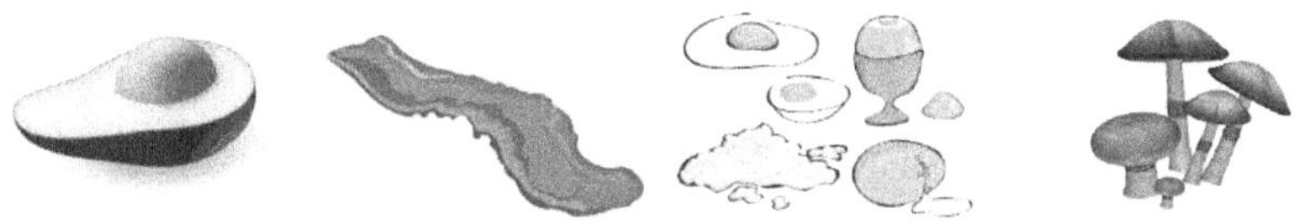

# Recipe 04: Breakfast Salad

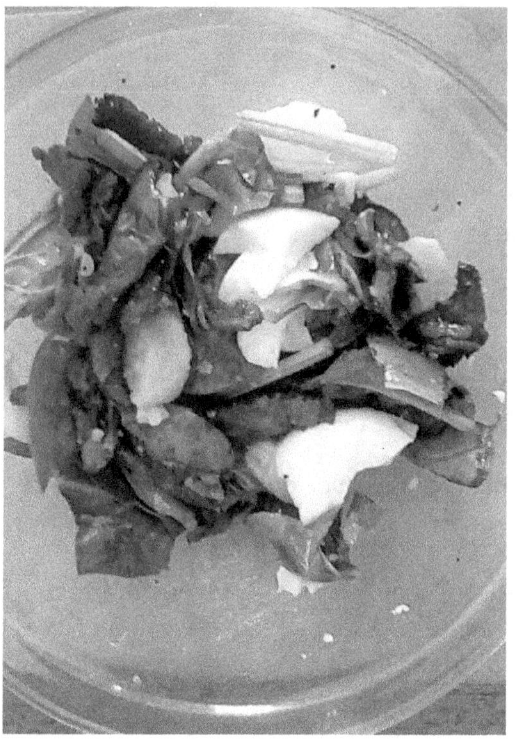

**INGREDIENTS:**

- Boiled eggs
- Bacon
- bibb lettuce or baby spinach leaves
- oil
- apple cider vinegar
- salt and pepper

Combine crumbled crispy bacon, chopped boiled eggs, lettuce or spinach in a bowl. Add 1 T. oil, 1 t. apple cider vinegar, salt and pepper to approximately one cup of lettuce. Toss well.

# Recipe 05: Breakfast Sausage

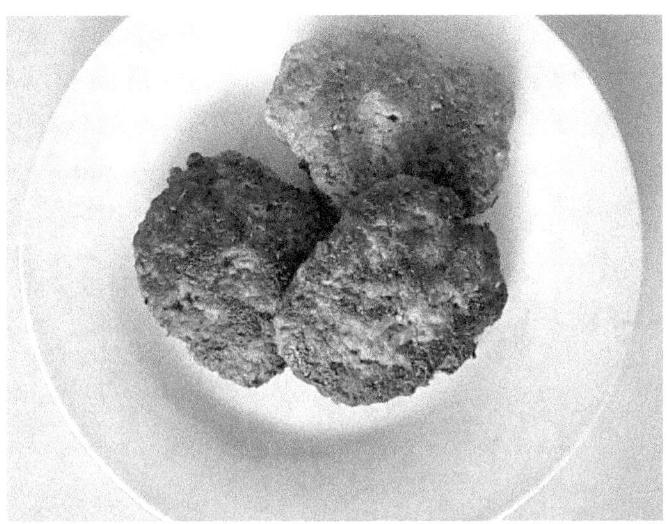

**INGREDIENTS**:

- ½  lb ground pork (in Styrofoam tray)
- 1 t. salt
- 2 T. sage
- 1 t. thyme
- ½ t. garlic powder
- ¼ t. onion powder
- 1 t. cumin
- 1 t. lemon pepper
- ½ t. Black Pepper
- 1 T. Oil

1. Use ground pork that has not been frozen.
2. Mix your seasonings in a small bowl first; then add seasonings to the ground pork. Mix very well.
3. Form your breakfast patties or simply brown in a skillet for loose meat. Make patties or links ahead to save time!

# Recipe 06: Cauliflower Hash Brown Fry Up

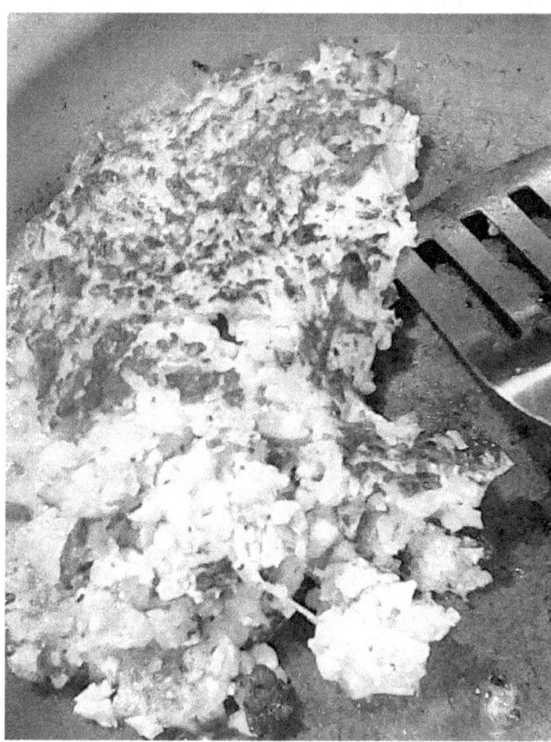

I cannot stress out good this is! It taste very much like traditional potato hash browns so this is something I feel certain you and your family will like!

**INGREDIENTS**:

- 1 cup riced cauliflower (from fresh, raw cauliflower)
- 1 strip crispy bacon, crumbled
- ¼ cup diced onion
- 1 whole egg

1. Combine riced cauliflower, cooked bacon, onion, egg, salt and pepper.

2. Heat 2 T. oil in a skillet.
3. Press the cauliflower mixture into the skillet and allow it to brown on one side without turning or stirring. Cook on medium heat.
4. Check the bottom for browning after a few minutes or so. Once you see a solid browning then you should be able to flip the cauliflower over to brown the other side. Don't worry that it may break apart because you will ultimately stir it into itself like you would hash browns anyway.

Comments:……………………………………………

………………………………………………………………………

………………………………………………………………………

………………………………………………………………………

*According to Mercola.com, among other well respected sites:*

*[Cauliflower is a member of the cancer-fighting cruciferous family of vegetables. Cauliflower is anti-inflammatory and antioxidant-rich, and may boost both your heart and brain health.*
*Eating cauliflower will provide your body with impressive amounts of vitamin C, vitamin k, beta-carotene, and much more while supporting healthy digestion and detoxification.]*

# Recipe 07: Drop Biscuits

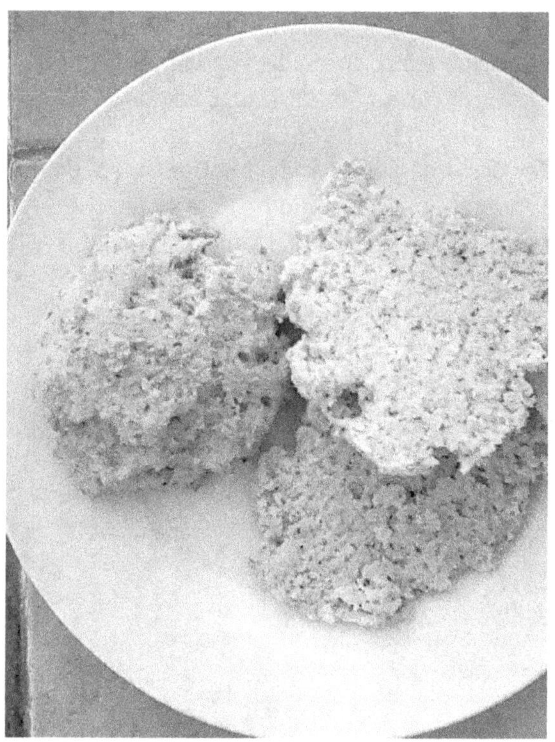

**INGREDIENTS:**

- 1 cup Almond flour
- 1 t. baking powder
- ½ t. salt
- 2 T. Gluten Free Bisquick
- 1 t. Xanthan Gum
- 1 whole large egg (not extra-large)
- ¾ ounce melted real unsalted butter, or refined coconut oil (without the coconut flavor)
- 3 T. hot water
- ½ t. apple cider vinegar

**Instructions**:

1.  Place all dry ingredients in a large bowl. Stir.
2.  In a smaller bowl, combine: egg, melted oil and the hot water.
3.  Mix the wet ingredients with the dry ingredients. Stir loosely.
4.  Add the apple cider vinegar. Mix well with a spoon, but do not over mix.
5.  Drop your standard size biscuits using a spoon, onto a greased baking sheet. This recipe makes about 4 biscuits. You could also put these in a muffin tin.
6.  Bake in a 350 degree **preheated** oven for about 20-25 minutes. Biscuits should be a golden brown. Check the bottoms. If you find soft spots, they are not done yet.

Comments:…………………………………………

………………………………………………………………………………

………………………………………………………………………………

………………………………………………………………………………

# Recipe 08: Egg Muffins

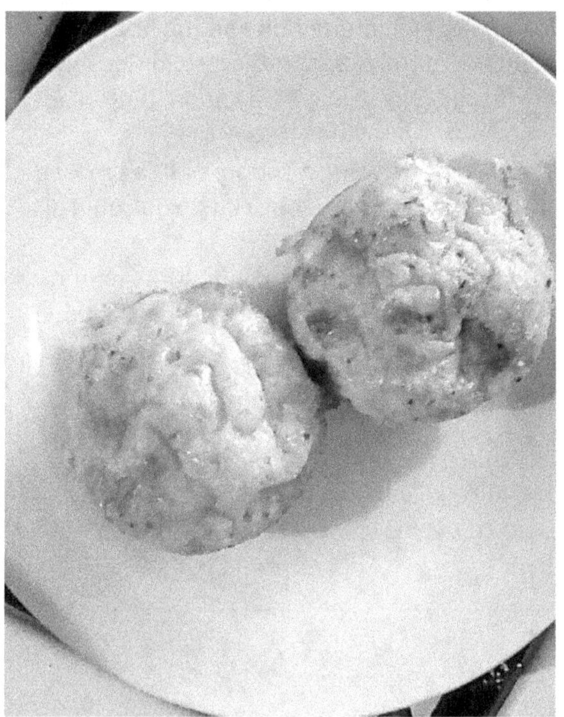

**INGREDIENTS**:

- 1 cup prepared breakfast sausage, Recipe 05: Breakfast Sausage
- ~double the black pepper for more heat
- 6 eggs

1. Preheat oven to 350 degrees.
2. Whisk the eggs, salt and pepper in a glass or stainless steel bowl.
3. Combine the eggs and prepared sausage.
4. Spray a muffin tin with nonstick cooking spray.
5. Using a 1/3 cup measuring cup as a serving, measure out one serving for each of the muffin cups.
6. This should just make 6 muffins.

7.     Bake at 350 degrees for about 20 minutes. Muffins should rise and be turning a golden brown around the edges. Allow the muffins to cool about 15 minutes before trying to remove. Use a butter knife or fork to loosen around the sides. These reheat well so make them ahead for the week.

Comments:……………………………………………

………………………………………………………………………………………………………

………………………………………………………………………………………………………

………………………………………………………………………………………………………

# Recipe 09: Egg on Top Breakfast Stack

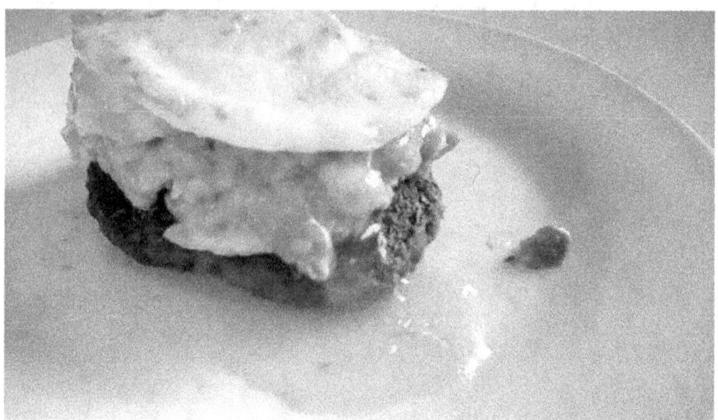

## INGREDIENTS:

- 2 homemade cooked breakfast patties: Recipe 05
- Use an egg ring if you want to be sure your patties and the eggs are the same size for easier stacking.
- 2 eggs
- 1 ripe avocado

## INSTRUCTIONS:

1. Cook your breakfast patties if you haven't already. Plate.
2. Mash avocado and scoop on top of patty
3. In a skillet fry your eggs to your liking. Over easy is nice because it allows for the runny yoke when you cut into it!
4. Place your egg on top!

# Recipe 10: Egg salad Sandwich

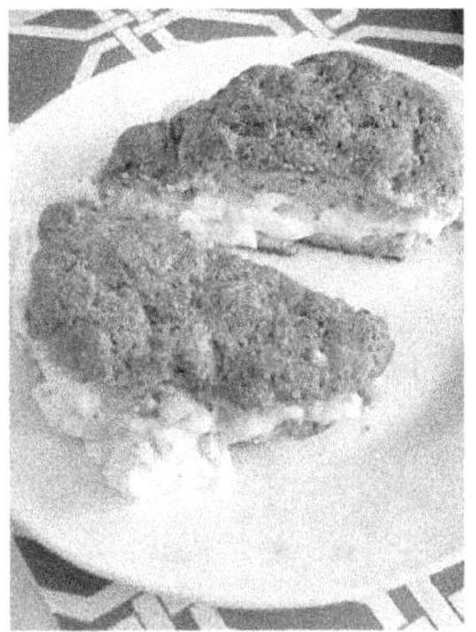

Egg salad is perfect for breakfast because you can make it over the weekend or the night before. You can also eat it without any bread, or use a low carb tortilla or a gluten free bread or biscuit, or even toast. This egg salad also pairs nicely with fresh spinach for lunch.

INGREDIENTS:

- 2 Boiled eggs (mix while the yolks are still warm)
- 3 T. mayo
- 1 t. Dijon mustard
- 2 T. diced celery
- 1/8 t celery seed
- Salt and pepper

Place eggs in cold water completely submerged. Bring to a full boil. Remove from heat. Cover. Wait 15 minutes. Peel, chop eggs coarsely, add to mixture of: mayo, mustard, celery, and seasonings.

Egg salad makes a nice sandwich for breakfast, lunch, or supper. You can also ditch the bread and instead use the egg salad as a dip with your Sunflower Seed Crackers Recipe 65, or in a healthy, low carb tortilla for a take-on-the-go wrap. I must admit that my favorite thing to do with egg salad is to place it on top a nice lettuce salad!

Comments:………………………………………………………

………………………………………………………………………………

………………………………………………………………………………

# Recipe 11: English Muffin

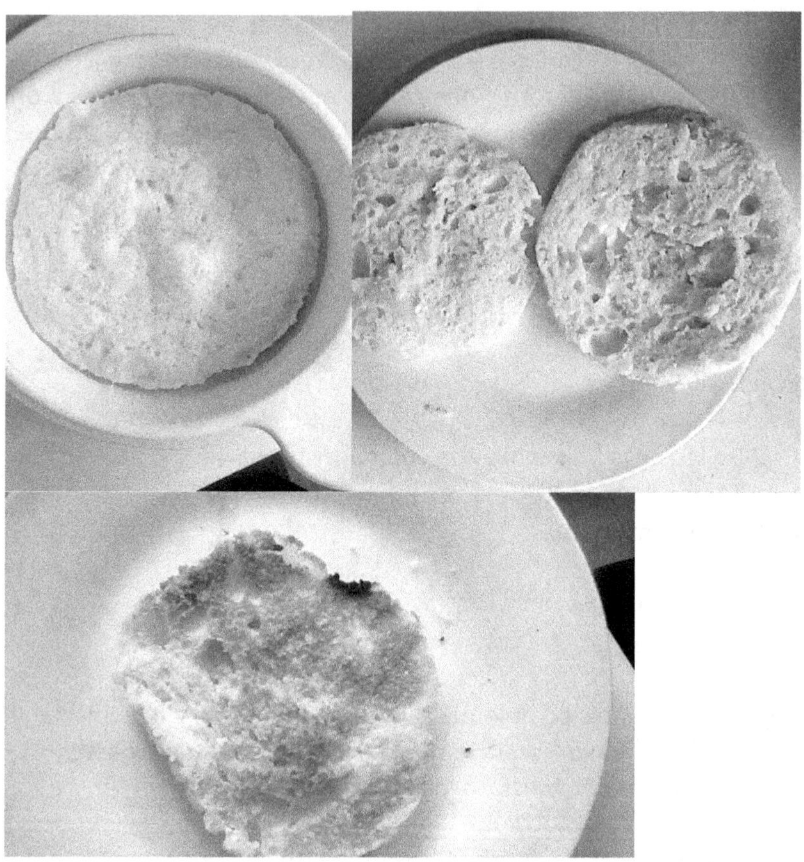

**INGREDIENTS**

- 3 T. almond flour
- 1 t. coconut flour
- 1 t. solid butter, ghee or coconut oil, melted
- 1 large egg
- A pinch of salt
- ½ t. baking powder

## INSTRUCTIONS:

1. Mix all ingredients in a bowl. Mix well. Do not replace solid fat with an oil. Be sure it is a solid fat that you melt, then add to the rest of the ingredients.
2. Pour into a microwavable safe dish (at least 4 inches in diameter with flat bottom recommended) or, an oven proof dish with sides if baking in the oven.
3. Allow to sit until "set". About 2 full minutes.

4. Microwave for 90 seconds exactly. Or, bake in a preheated 350 degree oven for 15 minutes.

5. Turn out onto a plate. Slice in half and THEN toast in toaster, toaster oven or back in the oven until a toasty brown.

This is dry but presumably you will use it as a vessel for some other food, such as a sausage patty, an egg, butter and berries. Has a cornmeal or Triscuit like texture to it.

Comments:…………………………………………

……………………………………………………………………………………

……………………………………………………………………………………

……………………………………………………………………………………

# Recipe 12: Fried Portabella and Eggs

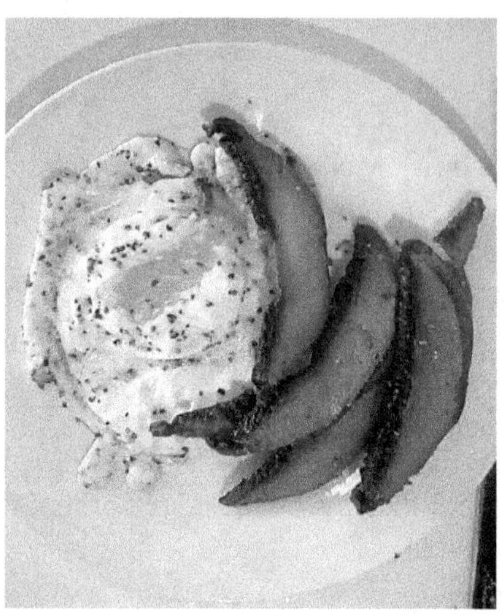

**INGREDIENTS**:

- Portabella Mushroom, sliced
- 1 egg
- Oil, salt and pepper

INSTRUCTIONS:

1. Coat the bottom of a cold skillet with oil, salt and pepper. Remember that mushrooms absorb some of the oil so while you do not want them swimming, you do want enough to still have some oil covering the bottom of the skillet.
2. Heat to a medium heat. Then add mushroom slices coating both sides and then allowing to fry on one side to a golden brown before turning.
3. Fry slices of mushroom until tender and golden brown. About 15 minutes.
4. You can then prepare your eggs whatever way you choose, fried, scrambled, poached, hard-boiled, or an omelet.

# Recipe 13: Fruit and Unsalted Nuts

Sometimes breakfast is more about ideas then full on recipes. Anytime you can eat whole fresh, unprocessed foods and feel satisfied is a victory for your health!
We all love our fruit but it can be a high carb food. Limit portions if you eat any at all and choose wisely.
There is a website I like to use to check carb counts of foods: twofoods.com I am not affiliated with them in any way but I use this site a lot. Pay attention to the portion size as well as the carb count. You can also check carb counts on fatsecret's website. Some common fruits with their respective carb counts:

**Mango** has a whopping 28 carbs per one cup of fruit

One medium size **pear** has about 25 carbs, as does a medium **banana**

An **orange** has about 15 carbs

**Blackberries**: per one cup has about 12 carbs

**Strawberries**: per one cup has about 12 carbs

**Watermelon**, per one cup servings: 12 carbs

Choose a **tangerine** (instead of an orange) and get just 9 carbs

**Peaches** average about 9 carbs per medium size fruit.

One average size **plum** has 7 carbs

One **Apricot** has just 4 carbs!

# Recipe 14: Pancakes (basic)

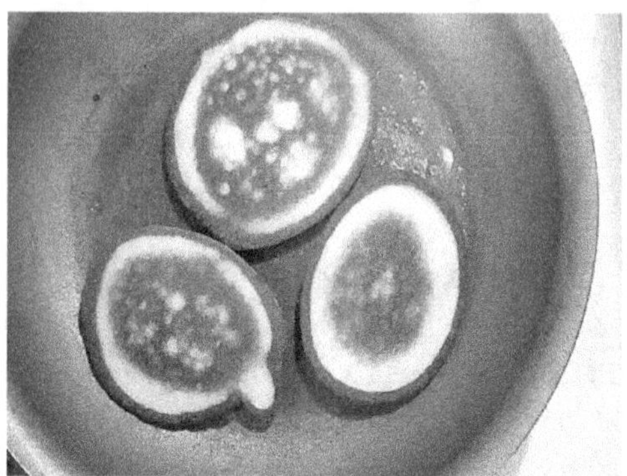

**INGREDIENTS**

Looking for a No-flour Pancake? See Recipe 16 in the Breakfast chapter

- 1 cup Almond flour
- ¼ cup water
- 2 large eggs (not extra large eggs)
- 1 t. raw, unfiltered honey or ½ t. sugar
- Coconut Oil for the skillet or a nonstick cooking spray

1 teaspoon of honey has about 7 carbs while ½ teaspoon white sugar has about 2). *This makes about six 4 inch pancakes* which gives you a total carb (including the almond flour) of 7 carbs per pancake. By comparison, a wheat flour pancake of the same size would have 16 carbs.

Combine all ingredients using a fork until eggs have combined well. Make as you normally would a pancake. I encourage you to try this basic recipe first. Taste it. Then decide if you want to add optional ingredients like vanilla, cinnamon, nuts, and or berries the next time you make it or with the remaining batter. This makes a nice sandwich with the Breakfast Sausage Recipe 05 too. Likewise, you could add some water to the batter, thinning it out, and make crepes.

Easily make this a savory pancake for lunch or supper by adding sliced scallions.

# Recipe 15: Mushroom and Zucchini Frittata

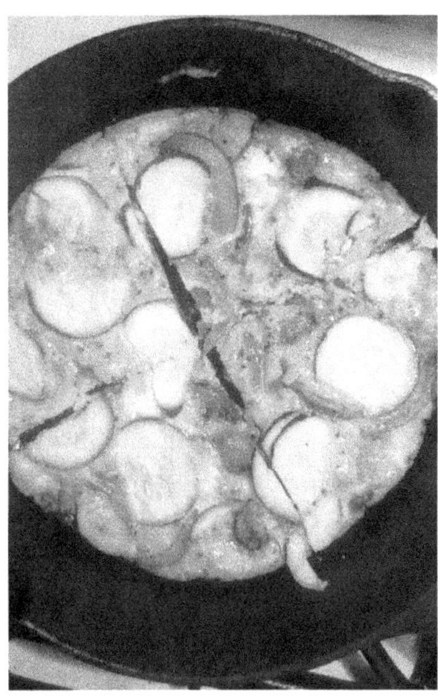

A Frittata can absolutely be made ahead, refrigerated and heated up or eaten cold or even room temperature!

## INGREDIENTS:

- 2 large eggs
- 4 ounces thinly sliced mushrooms
- Shaved zucchini ( I use the side slicer on my grater for nice very thin slices)
- 2 tablespoons diced onion
- Salt and pepper
- Oven proof skillet

**INSTRUCTIONS:**

1. Preheat oven to 400 degrees
2. Toss the mushrooms, onion, oil, salt and pepper in a bowl.
3. Saute' mushrooms until starting to turn a toasty brown.
4. Whisk your eggs and pour evenly over the mushrooms. Be sure you still have the skillet over medium to high heat.
5. Cook on the stove top for a minute or two until you see the eggs starting to set on the edges of your skillet.
6. Spread your shaved zucchini evenly over the top of the eggs.
7. Bake at 400 degrees in preheated oven for about 10 minutes.
8. Allow your frittata to sit and rest for 5-10 minutes after removing from the oven before slicing or eating.

Comments:..............................................

...............................................................................................

...............................................................................................

# Recipe 16: No-Flour Pancake

INGREDIENTS:

- ½ cup cooked pumpkin
- 2 eggs
- 2 T. coconut oil (solid, not the liquid) or, Unsalted Real Butter.

INSTRUCTIONS:

Place all ingredients in your blender or food processor and blend until you have a smooth batter.

Cook these a bit slower than you would a traditional pancake to ensure they cook through. Cook about 7 minutes on the first side before flipping.

Walnuts, vanilla, and/or cinnamon in the batter is a nice optional addition to this recipe.

Comments:…………………………………………

……………………………………………………………………………………

……………………………………………………………………………………

……………………………………………………………………………………

# Recipe 17: Sausage Biscuit

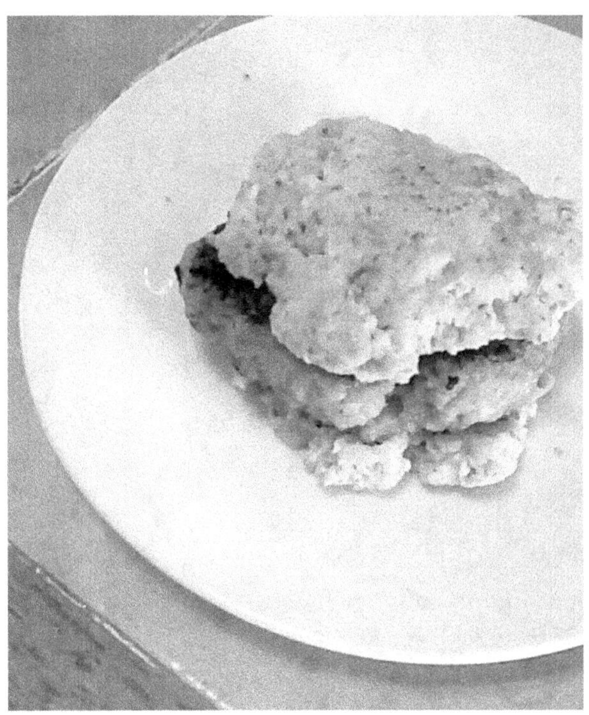

Drop Biscuit Recipe 07
Breakfast Sausage Recipe 05

Comments:...............................................

.................................................................................

.................................................................................

.................................................................................

# Recipe 18: Sausage Gravy

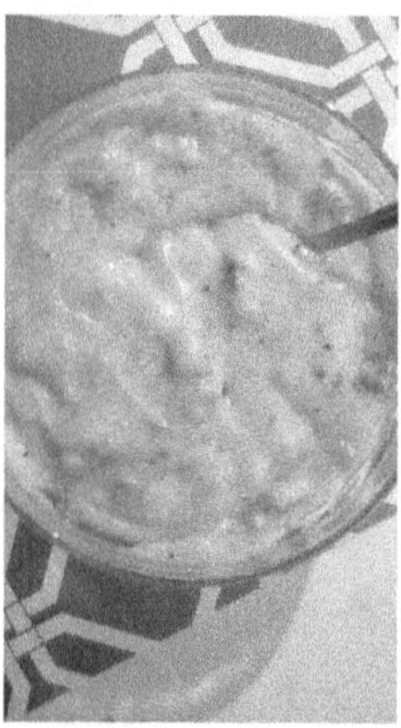

INGREDIENTS:

- ¼ lb Ground pork
- 2 T. gf flour (I tried almond flour, my favorite, but it does not work. So I used GF Bisquick)
- 1 Cup Almond Milk (Unsweetened Original which has just 1 carb per cup)
- 1 t. salt
- 2 T. sage
- 1 t. thyme
- ½ t. garlic powder
- ¼ t. onion powder
- 1 t. cumin
- 1 t. lemon pepper
- ½ t. Black Pepper

## INSTRUCTIONS:

1. Brown pork in a skillet over medium to high heat. Add seasonings and flour and whisk immediately to blend until smooth.
2. Add milk and continue to whisk. You may want to turn the heat down a bit.
3. Will thicken within minutes.

4. You could also use this recipe for chicken gravy with fried chicken fat after removing the chicken from the skillet.

*2 T. of GF Bisquick has 12 carbs. This recipe makes 2 servings (1/2 c. each) so you will get approximately 6 carbs per serving. You can use regular all-purpose flour of course if you do not avoid gluten but, all-purpose flour has about 22 carbs per 2 Tablespoons. (2 tablespoons equals 1 ounce)*

Comments:…………………………………………

…………………………………………………………………………………

…………………………………………………………………………………

…………………………………………………………………………………

## LUNCH AND SUPPER RECIPES:

# 78 LUNCH AND SUPPER RECIPES

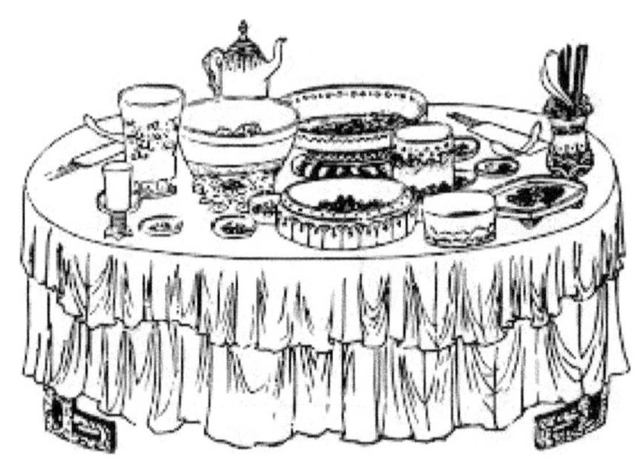

# Recipe 01: Alfredo Sauce

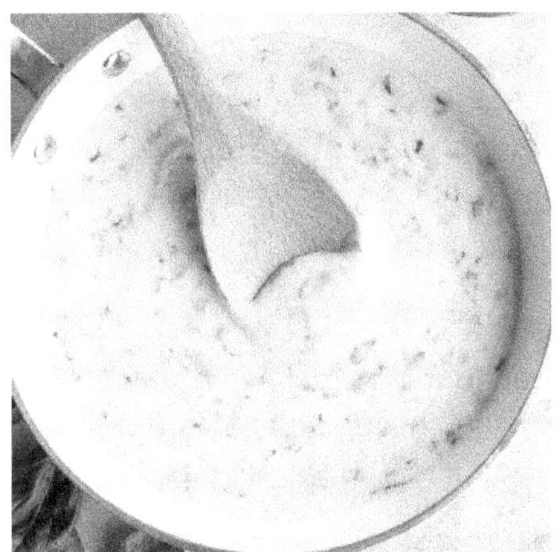

INGREDIENTS

- ¾ cup Almond Milk, Unflavored Original
- 2 T. oil
- 2 T. cornstarch
- ¾ cup chicken broth
- 1 tsp garlic powder
- ½ tsp lemon pepper
- ½ tsp onion powder
- 2 T. chopped fresh parsley

**INSTRUCTIONS**

1. Heat oil in skillet. Whisk in cornstarch stirring until a smooth paste. Add milk stirring constantly. Should thicken almost immediately. Begin to add broth until the consistency you like.
2. Add seasonings except parsley. Cover and let simmer about 15 minutes.
3. Add parsley once you have removed from heat.

## Recipe 02: Asian Dressing

**INGREDIENTS**

- 2 T. oil
- 3 T. Soy Sauce or Coconut Aminos if you are avoiding soy
- 3 T. Rice Wine Vinegar
- 1 T. Lemon Juice
- 1 T. Sesame Seed Oil
- Salt and Pepper

Mix all. Taste, and adjust ingredients for your taste palate. When making dressings like this one I like to place the ingredients in a glass jar, place the lid on and shake it up to combine the ingredients.

Comments:……………………………………………

………………………………………………………………………

………………………………………………………………………

………………………………………………………………………

# Recipe 03: Asian Slaw

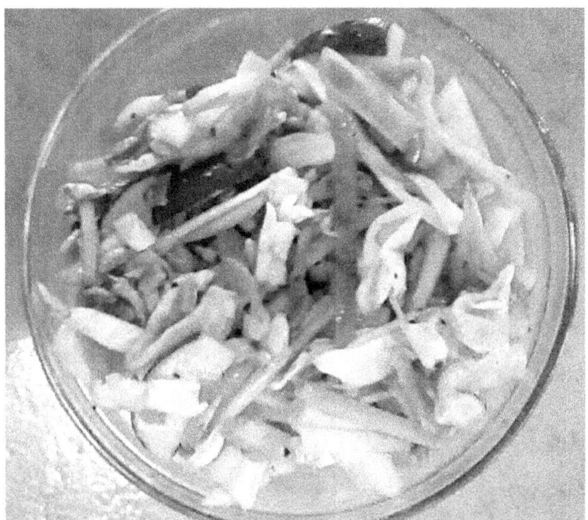

Asian Slaw uses the Asian Dressing Recipe 02

## INGREDIENTS

- ¼ cup snow peas, sliced into strips
- 2 large radishes, sliced into matchstick strips
- ¼ c celery, matchstick strips
- 1 cup cabbage of choice or mix a couple (white cabbage, Chinese cabbage, red cabbage) sliced into strips
- ¼ cup grated (shredded) carrots; about one small carrot
- Sunflower Seeds (optional)

## INSTRUCTIONS:

1. Make the Asian Dressing, Recipe 02 and set aside.
2. In a medium bowl combine all of vegetables.
3. Pour the dressing over the cabbage mixture and toss to coat.
4. A handful of sunflower seeds or sliced pecans is a nice addition to this salad.

# Recipe 04: Asparagus Salad

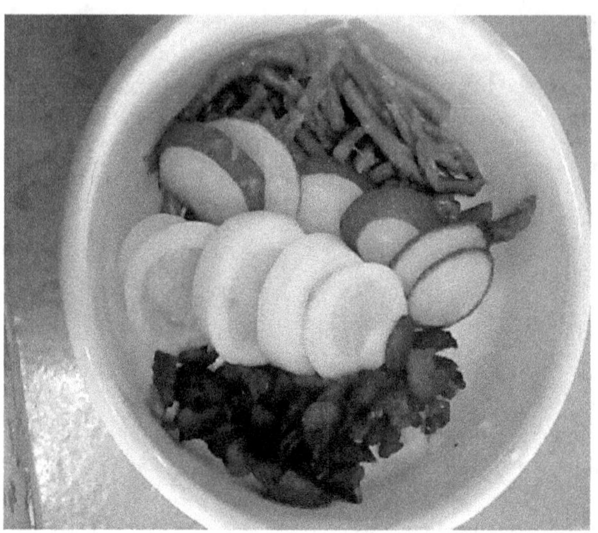

**INGREDIENTS**

- Asparagus in bite size pieces (cooked and chilled)
- Radishes, chopped
- Boiled egg, chopped or sliced
- Bacon, crispy and crumbled
- Lemon Vinaigrette Recipe 46

A great cold salad generally made from leftovers! Just mix all the ingredients together.

# Recipe 05: Asparagus Soup

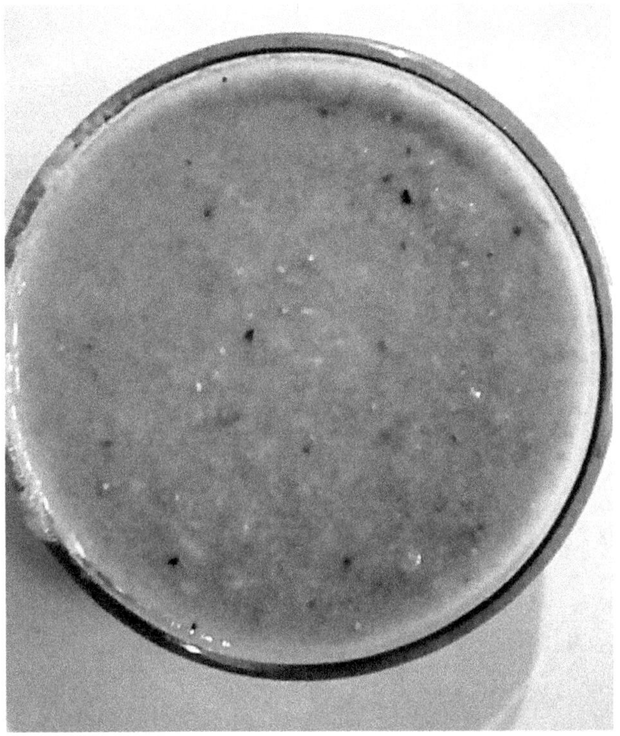

## INGREDIENTS

- ½ cup chicken stock or broth
- 2 T.  lemon juice
- 1 ½ cups cooked asparagus
- Salt and pepper

## INSTRUCTIONS

Combine all ingredients in your blender and blend until smooth. Taste and adjust seasonings and lemon juice if desired. This soup is good room temperature, cold, or hot.

# Recipe 06: Baked Portabella Mushrooms

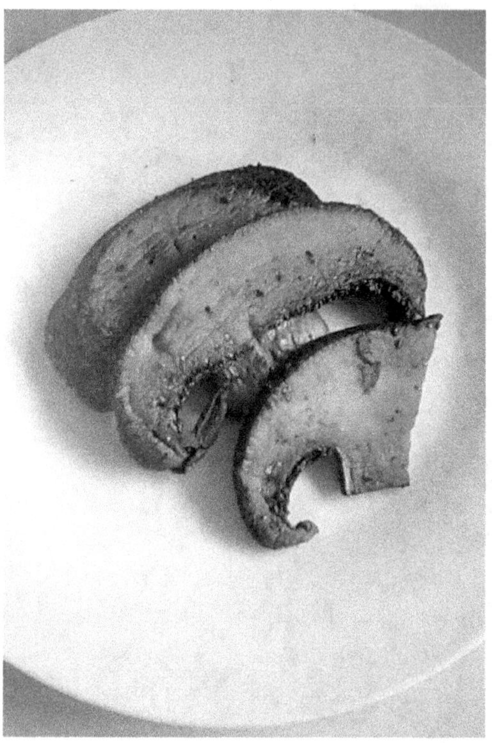

**INGREDIENTS**

- Sliced Portabella mushrooms
- Oil
- Salt and Pepper

Heat oven to 400 degrees. Toss mushrooms in a bowl with oil, salt and pepper until thoroughly coated. Pour all, including excess oil onto baking sheet. Spread mushrooms to even layer. Bake about 15-20 minutes until turning a golden brown. Turn over. Cook an additional 5 minutes.

These are great with eggs for breakfast, on a turkey burger or as its own vegan burger! Serve with pesto like you might eggplant if you are avoiding nightshades.

# Recipe 07: Basic White Sauce

**INGREDIENTS**

- 1 T. butter of choice or your favorite healthy oil
- 2 T. gf flour (I tried almond flour, my favorite and it does not work. So I used GF Bisquick: 6 carbs/serving)
- 1 Cup Almond Milk (Unsweetened Original which has just 1 carb per cup)

1. Heat butter or fat in a skillet over medium to high heat. Add flour and whisk immediately to blend until smooth.
2. Add milk and continue to whisk. You may want to turn the heat down a bit.
3. Will thicken within minutes.

4. You could also use this recipe for chicken gravy with fried chicken. Use the fat rendered after removing your chicken from the skillet.

2 T. of GF Bisquick has 12 carbs. This recipe makes 2 servings (1/2 c. each) so you will get approximately 6 carbs per serving. You can use regular all-purpose flour of course if you do not avoid gluten but, all-purpose flour has about 22 carbs per 2 Tablespoons. (2 tablespoons equals 1 ounce)

# Recipe 08: Beef Shank Roast n Vegetables

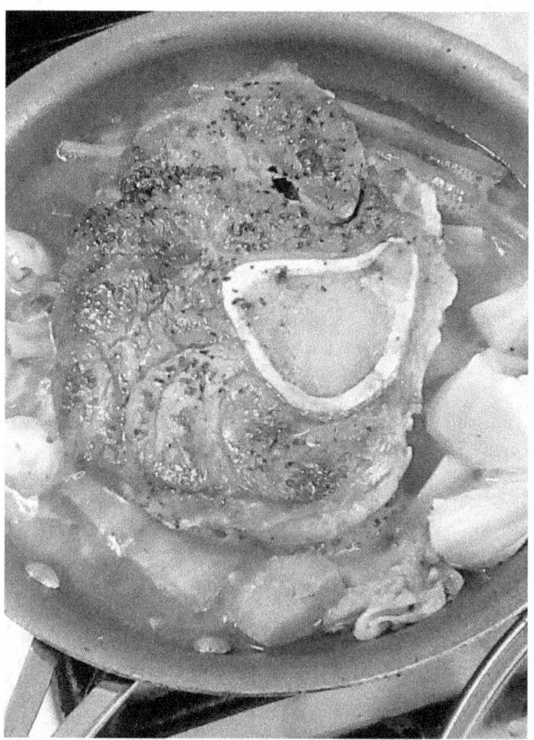

**INGREDIENTS**

- 2 Beef shanks bone-in
- 1 cup chicken or beef broth
- 1 cup water
- 2 medium carrots
- 1 stalk celery
- 1 small onion
- 1 (8oz) pkg mushrooms
- 2 T cornstarch (optional if you want gravy)

INSTRUCTIONS:

1. Brown thawed shanks until golden brown on both sides turning just once.
2. Add broth and scrape bottom of pan. Add water. Liquid should come up just halfway on the shanks. The beef shanks should not be covered. It should look more like you are going to poach them, not boil them.
3. Crock Pot method: place vegetables in the bottom of the crock pot. After browning shanks in a skillet on both sides, add browned shanks to crock pot on top of the vegetables, then add liquid. Do not put so much liquid that your beef is submerged in liquid. Do make sure the vegetables are covered in broth. Sprinkle salt and pepper and thyme on top of shanks. Cover and cook in crock pot 3 hours on high or 6 hours on low.

Skillet Method:

1. After browning both sides of shanks, add liquid. Bring to a high simmer and cover. Cook one hour. Add vegetables, cover, and continue to cook another 2 hours or until meat is tender (should easily separate from bone) and vegetables are tender.
2. Gravy: make a slurry with one ladle of stock/drippings and the cornstarch. Using a whisk, add in remaining broth, over medium to high heat, until well blended. Cook until thickened, just a few minutes.

*A slurry is when you take a binder like cornstarch, flour or arrowroot and blend it with a small amount of broth or liquid until smooth. Then, whisk it into the remaining broth or liquid to thicken it up.*

*Cornstarch has 9 carbs per Tablespoon. Spread out over this gravy which should provide approximately 3-6 people will bring the carb count to about 3 carbs or less. Arrowroot is a good alternative for those avoiding cornstarch.*

# Recipe 09: Blonde Chicken and Gravy

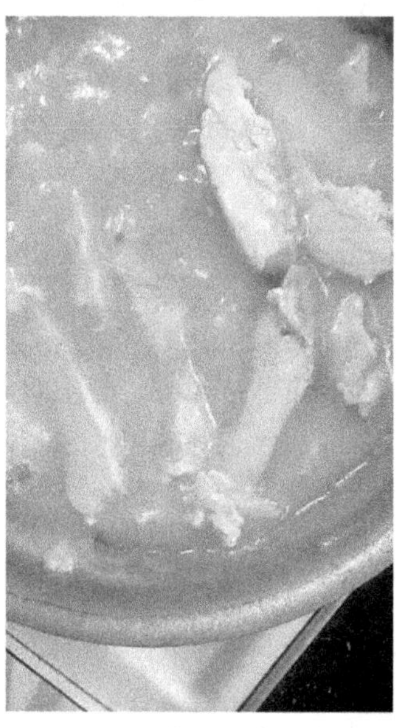

**INGREDIENTS**

- 2 chicken breasts
- 4 cups chicken broth
- 4 T. Real, Unsalted Butter or your non-dairy preference
- 4 T. Gluten Free Bisquick
- Salt and Pepper
- 3 T. oil

**INSTRUCTIONS**

1. Rub your chicken breasts in the oil, salt and pepper. Brown on both sides in hot skillet. A nice golden brown. About 5 minutes on both sides.
2. Add broth to skillet making sure to NOT completely cover the chicken. We want to poach the chicken in the broth, not boil it.
3. Cover and simmer 20 minutes.
4. Remove the chicken from the skillet to a plate to rest.
5. Remove the broth to a bowl.
6. Add the butter to the skillet and then the flour to make a roux. Be sure to stir constantly and when the roux is smooth and free of lumps start to add the broth back into the skillet using a whisk.
7. The broth should thicken quite quickly. Continue adding broth until you feel it is at the consistency you like for a gravy or sauce.
8. Add the chicken back to the skillet. Sometimes I will go ahead and slice the chicken, shred it or you can also leave it as is.
9. You are ready to serve your blonde Chicken and Gravy!

# Recipe 10: Boiled Spaghetti Squash

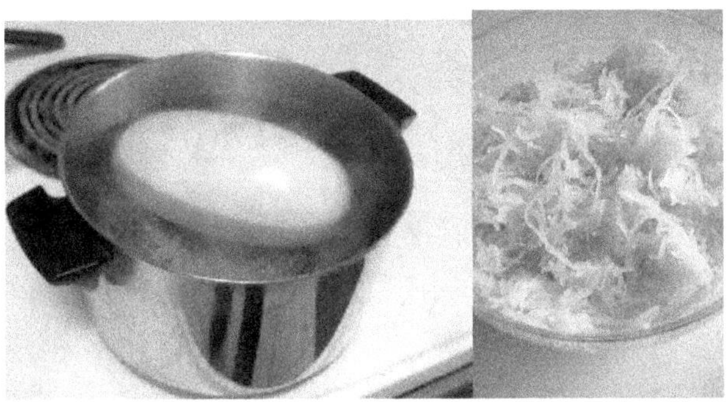

**INGREDIENTS**:

- Whole spaghetti squash
- 6 quart (minimum) stock pot
- 5 quarts of water
- Salt, pepper, oil
- 1 tsp minced garlic and 1 tsp minced basil or Italian seasoning

INSTRUCTIONS:

1. Place your raw, whole spaghetti squash into the stock pot. Fill with water. Boil until you can puncture the rind of the squash easily with a paring knife. About an hour or so depending on the size of your squash.
2. Remove from water and allow to cool about 30 minutes. Cut the ends off and then cut in half. Using an ice cream scoop, remove the seeds.
3. You should be able to easily remove the skin from the squash. Discard.
4. Place the cooked squash in a large glass bowl and toss (to loosen up and separate) the squash noodle.
5. Toss the noodles with oil, salt, pepper, basil and garlic. Place in shallow baking dish. Cover and bake at 400 degrees for about 15 minutes to heat up and allow the basil and garlic to marry with the oil.

# Recipe 11: Bread Rolls (for sandwiches and buns)

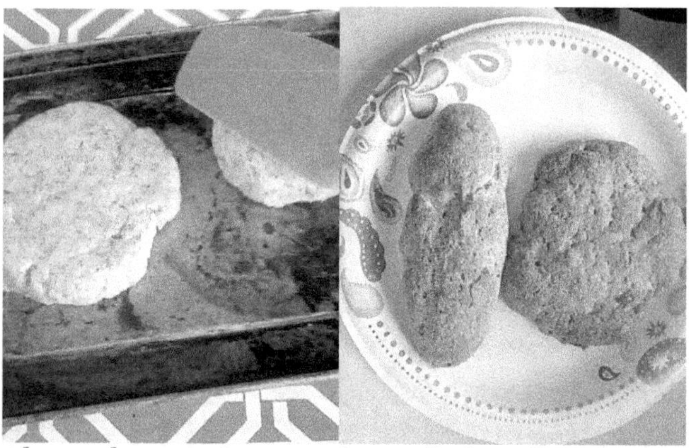

Also makes an nice crunchy garlic bread.

**INGREDIENTS**:

- *1 c. almond flour*
- *1 T. xanthan gum*
- *2 T. Gluten Free Bisquick*
- *1 t. baking powder*
- *¼ tsp salt*
- *2 t. oil*
- *1 egg white*
- *1 whole egg*
- *1 t. ACV*
- *1 T. warm water*

1. Place almond flour, baking powder, xanthan gum, gf Bisquick, and salt together.
2. In another small bowl, whisk the eggs, oil. (you will add the vinegar and water later)
3. Add to flour.
4. Then...... add the apple cider vinegar.
5. Now add the water and combine well. Forming into a ball. Dough will feel wet.

6.  Let the dough sit about 20 minutes. Then work the dough once more. The dough will still feel wetter than a traditional bread dough.

7.  Bake at 350 for 20 minutes, or until golden on the outside and cooked thoroughly inside.

This bread is quite dense. For some sandwiches you may want to hollow out the bread before adding contents. Also makes a nice crusty bread when put back into the oven later in the week.

Elevation and humidity can affect the outcome of this recipe.

Comments:…………………………………………

……………………………………………………………………………

……………………………………………………………………………

……………………………………………………………………………

# Recipe 12: Buttery Garlic Cabbage

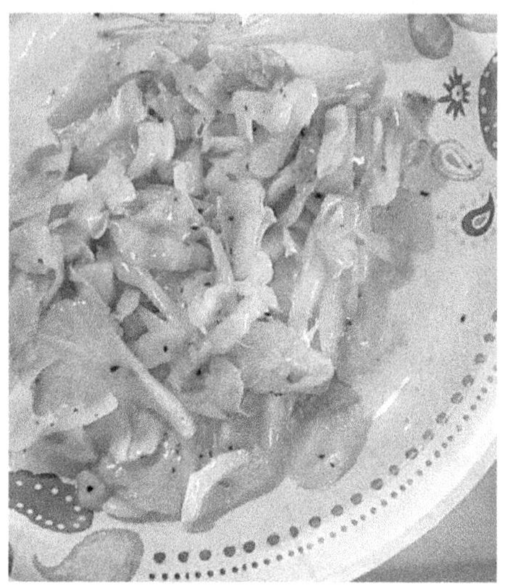

*This recipe uses butter. As with any recipe, you can always substitute your own oil or butter alternative. I find Avocado oil is a nice substitute for the butter in this dish.*

INGREDIENTS:

- ½ medium head white cabbage
- 4-6 tablespoons unsalted real butter and 1 T. Oil
- Salt and lemon pepper to taste

INSTRUCTIONS

1. Core the cabbage and slice it into thin strips.
2. Put your oil, butter, salt, and lemon pepper in a cold skillet. Heat to medium heat.
3. Add the strips of cabbage. Stir to coat.
4. Continue cooking and stirring occasionally until the cabbage is "al dente" or until it is green and tender without being mushy. You should be cooking over medium to high heat. Should take just 3.5 minutes.

# Recipe 13: Cauliflower "potato" Pancakes

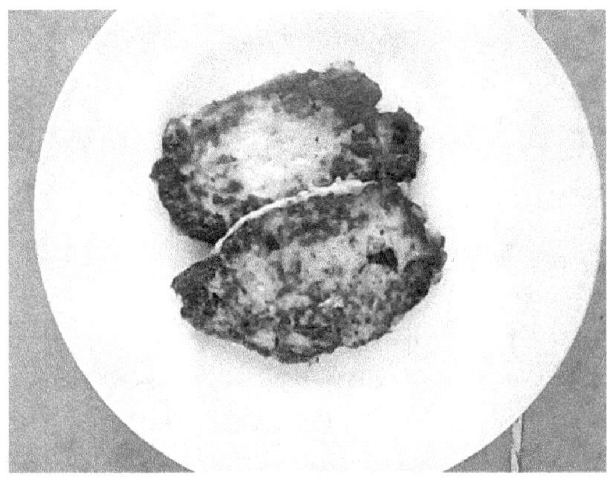

You can start from a fresh head of cauliflower or use leftover Mashed Cauliflower Recipe 47.

INGREDIENTS:

- 1 head small cauliflower
- 2 T extra virgin olive oil or real, unsalted butter
- 1 dash salt and dash of pepper to taste
- 1 t. onion powder
- 1 large egg

INSTRUCTIONS:

[If you are using leftover Mashed Cauliflower just add onion powder and the egg to your leftover mashed cauliflower.]

1. Chop cauliflower. Boil until *very* tender (about 15 minutes or so)
2. Drain well. I like to use my hand held masher and mash the cauliflower while in the strainer to get as much of the liquid out that I can.
3. Scoop the cauliflower into your bowl and add salt, pepper, and onion powder.
4. The addition of the egg should thin out your cauliflower mixture enough to drop into your skillet to make your pancakes. If not, add a tablespoon of water.
5. Brown on both sides over medium heat.

# Recipe 14: Cauliflower and Vegetables

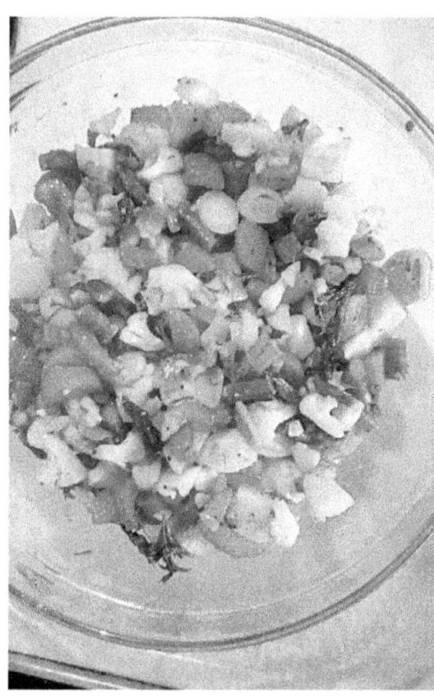

## INGREDIENTS:

- 1 tablespoon olive oil
- 1 celery stalk, diced
- 1 medium carrot, diced
- 1 garlic clove, minced
- 2 cups cauliflower "riced" or diced
- 4 Asparagus spears, chopped
- 2 Scallions chopped
- 2 T. chopped parsley
- Salt and Lemon Pepper

## Instructions

1. Heat the olive oil in a large deep skillet, and sauté the carrots and celery until they start to soften, about 5 minutes.
2. Add in the cauliflower and garlic with 1 T. water. Stir to combine. Stir occasionally and until starting to get tender.
3. Add asparagus. Cook 1-2 minutes.
4. Add parsley and chopped scallion after removing from heat.
5. Stir to coat.

Comments:...............................................

..................................................................

..................................................................

# Recipe 15: Chicken Broth

Save bones from whole hens. Backbone and from chicken legs, chicken wings, thighs and breasts. A backbone from a whole hen is enough to make broth on its own. For legs and wings from pieces I use a gallon size freezer bag and when it's about full I make broth. I keep a separate freezer bag in the freezer for beef bones until I have enough to make broth.
Place your bones in a stock pot or crock pot and fill with water. The only other thing I suggest adding is whole cloves of garlic but you can leave those out if you are not a fan of garlic. Not adding other ingredients will give you a wonderful pure broth that is delicious.
Allow to set at a high simmer for about 12 hours. Some of the water will evaporate so be sure you fill up your pot completely and check on occasion. Do not add more water though. Just add enough excess to allow for evaporation.
Allow to cool completely, uncovered, before placing in containers for the refrigerator or freezer.

You want to cool uncovered to minimize the possible growth of bacteria.

Homemade broth and stock can often times turn to a gelatin when refrigerated. That is collagen and perfectly safe, and in fact, very healthy for you to eat. When you heat that "gelatin" back up, it will return to a liquid broth.

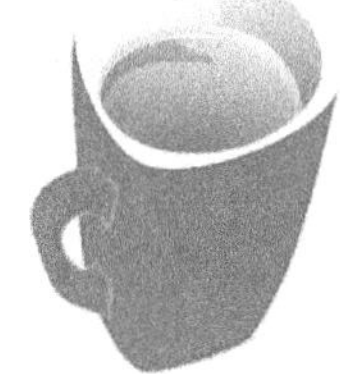

If you choose to use store bought broth on occasion please be sure to check out the ingredient label as well as the nutritional label.

What's the difference between stock and broth? Stock is made from boiling bones and broth is made from boiling just the meat. The stock will be a much richer and darker stock while broth made from boiling just meat without any bones will be a lighter more clear broth. Both are useful depending on your needs.

# Recipe 16: Chicken "Arti" Casserole

*If you are looking for a new Chicken Broccoli Casserole, I always get rave reviews when I make this!*

## INGREDIENTS

- 2-4 boneless chicken breast
- 1 ten ounce pkg frozen broccoli or equivalent fresh broccoli
- 1 (14 oz) can artichokes
- 1 egg
- 1 T. minced garlic
- 1 T. cornstarch or arrowroot
- 1 cup chicken broth
- Pinch or two of lemon pepper & Pinch of salt

## INSTRUCTIONS

1. Salt and pepper chicken breasts. Brown both sides (golden brown) in oven proof skillet or casserole dish.
2. Pour broth in skillet, over chicken. You may not use all of the broth. Only use enough to cover about halfway up the side of the chicken. You do not want to submerge it completely.
3. Bake in a 375 degree oven for 15 minutes.

While the chicken is baking:

- Drain can of artichokes and puree in chopper, blender or food processor with one egg and 1 T. cornstarch.
- In glass bowl combine pureed artichokes, broccoli, minced garlic, pinch of salt and lemon pepper.
- After chicken has baked the 15 minutes, remove from oven.
- Combine the broth just removed from oven with the broccoli and artichokes. Mix well.
- Pour the broccoli mixture over the chicken breasts.
- Place the chicken and broccoli back in the oven for 15 minutes if your chicken pieces are on the smaller side and about 20 minutes for large pieces.

# Recipe 17: Chicken Piccata

- 2 skinless and boneless chicken breasts, butterflied and then cut in half
- Cornstarch for sprinkling
- 2 tablespoons unsalted butter or oil
- 5 tablespoons extra-virgin olive oil
- ½ cup fresh lemon juice
- 2 cups chicken stock or 1 cup white wine and 1 cup chicken stock
- 1-2 ounces capers, drained and rinsed
- 2 large garlic cloves thinly sliced
- 2 T fresh parsley, chopped

**INSTRUCTIONS**

1. Combine the lemon juice, broth, capers, and garlic in a small glass bowl and set aside.

Traditionally, the chicken is pounded to thin cutlets before cooking. This makes for a delicate dish and the chicken will cook in just a few minutes.

Season chicken with salt and pepper, and sprinkle lightly with gf flour, cornstarch or arrowroot. (Cornstarch has the least carbs)

Heat oil in a large skillet over medium high heat. When oil starts to sizzle, add chicken and cook for about 3 minutes on one side. When chicken is browned, flip and cook other side for 3 minutes. Remove and transfer to a plate.

Into the skillet, add the lemon juice, stock, garlic and capers. Return to stove and bring to boil, scraping up brown bits from the pan for extra flavor. You may need to turn the heat down a bit. Check for seasoning/taste. Return the chicken to the pan and simmer for 5 minutes. Remove chicken to platter. Add butter to sauce and whisk vigorously. Pour sauce over chicken and garnish lightly with chopped parsley.

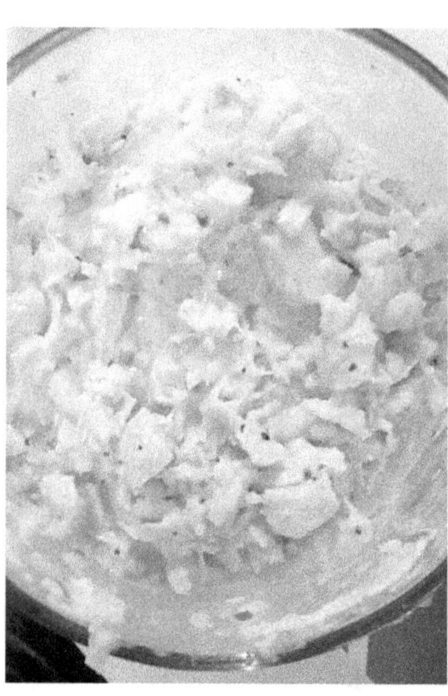

## Recipe 18: Chicken Salad

INGREDIENTS

- 1/3 cup diced celery (4 T.)
- 1/8 cup minced onion (2 T.)
- 2 T. Dill Pickle Relish
- 1 T. oil
- Salt and Pepper
- Healthy Mayo of choice (¼ cup)
- 2 cups cooked cold chicken

Mix all ingredients together well. Best after refrigerated for at least one hour. Will keep in refrigerator for 5 days.

## Recipe 19: Chicken Vegetable Soup

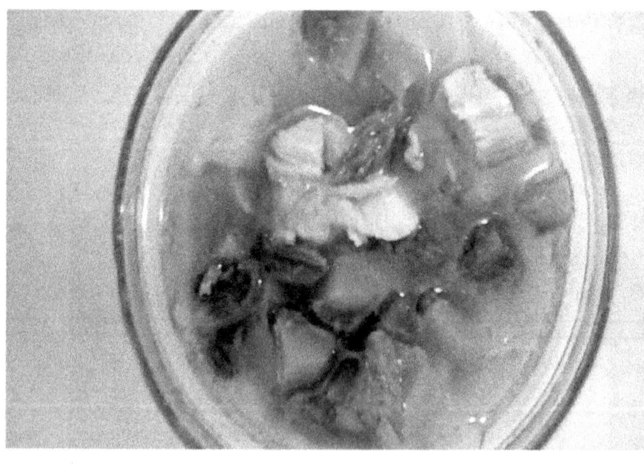

This is a wonderfully flavored soup you can make in under one hour.

*If you have never made your own chicken soup I hope you will give this a try and see* how much better it is than canned chicken soup, and also, that you don't need noodles in chicken soup for it to be a hearty, healing and comforting food.

- 1 ½ cups chicken broth
- ½ cup water
- 2 cups shredded or cubed leftover chicken (or, of course, 1 fresh chicken breast)

… if you have fresh chicken:

1. First brown chicken breasts on both sides in a bit of oil. About 5 minutes each side. Look for a nice golden browning. Chicken on the bone will give you a deeper tasting stock, while boneless chicken will give you a lighter more clear broth. Remove from skillet (chicken will finish cooking later)

2. Chop your vegetables into bite size pieces while chicken is cooking. Some low carb choices:
3. Green beans, celery, okra, mushrooms, snow peas, yellow squash, zucchini, carrot.

4. In a saucepan: add your vegetables to a bit of oil and sauté for just a minute or two. Add broth and water. Then add your seasonings:

5. Seasonings: I like to keep it traditional by using a bay leaf, thyme, garlic, sage.

6. Shred your chicken breasts or cut into bite size pieces and add to your broth and vegetables.
7. Bring to a boil. Cover and then lower heat to a simmer. Best when allowed to simmer for at least 30-60 minutes.

If you are going to make a batch of this to freeze I suggest only cooking about 15 minutes. Allow to cool completely uncovered before freezing. Also go ahead and remove the bay leaf before freezing.

# Recipe 20: Cilantro Lime Dip or Dressing

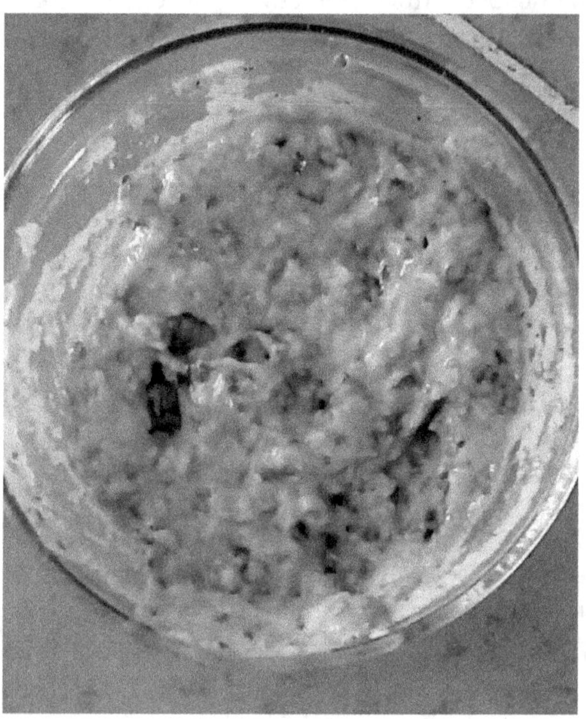

INGREDIENTS:

- ¾ cup chopped fresh cilantro
- 1 T.  red wine vinegar
- 1 dash salt
- 2 t. lime juice (or more per taste)
- 1/4 cup olive oil
- 2 garlic cloves
- 1/2 ripe avocado

Add all of your ingredients to your blender and blend just until smooth. Taste, adjust any ingredients. Best when chilled. For a thicker dip use less oil. For thinner dressing you want to pour, increase the oil and the lime juice in small increments until you get the consistency you want.

# Recipe 21: Cilantro Lime Riced Cauliflower

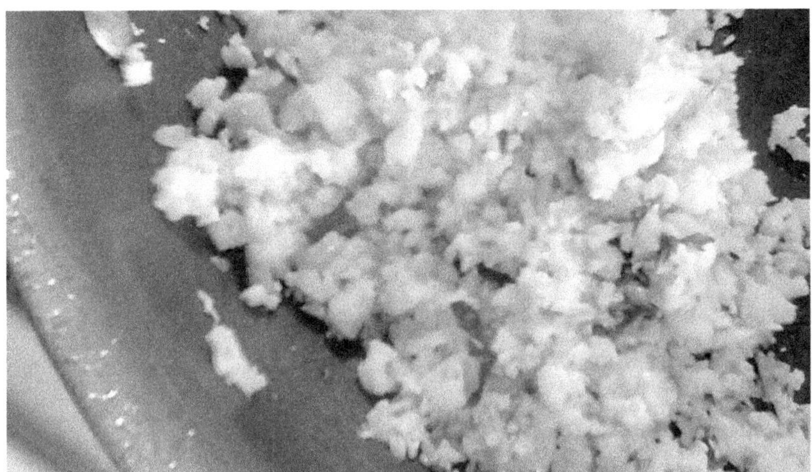

Also good using parsley instead of cilantro.

- ½ head riced cauliflower (using a knife or your chopper)
- ¼ cup oil
- ¼ cup chopped cilantro
- 2 large garlic cloves, minced
- 2 T. lime juice
- ¼ t. salt

1. Step one is to combine in a small bowl: oil, cilantro, garlic, salt, and lime juice. Set aside.
2. Step two is to chop (rice) your cauliflower.
3. Toss riced cauliflower with other ingredients. Allow to set at least 15 minutes.
4. Heat a skillet on high heat.
5. Spread the cauliflower evenly in the bottom of the skillet. Your mixture should not have excess oil. Just enough to thoroughly coat your cauliflower.

You are allowing the cauliflower to brown just a bit on the bottom. Takes about 5-7 minutes. Stir well in skillet. Remove from heat.

This is great by itself but also makes a nice side to fish and chicken.

## Recipe 22: Cobb Salad

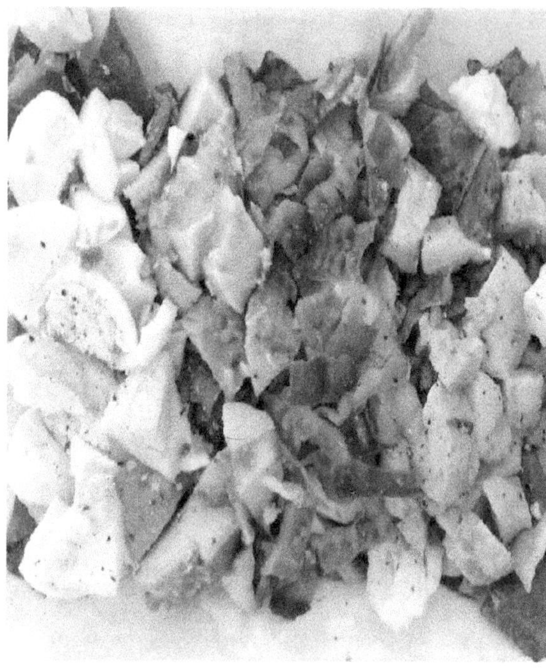

### Ingredients

- One cup chopped crisp lettuce like Romaine or Iceberg
- 1 large hard-boiled egg
- 2 ounces grilled chicken
- 2 1/2 slices bacon cooked and crumbled
- 1/2 ounce green onion about 1 large
- 1 ounce radish about 2 medium-large
- 1 1/2 ounces ripe avocado sliced
- Your favorite dressing

Arrange on a large plate or toss together in a bowl. Toss with your favorite dressing.

## Recipe 23: Cold Chopped Vegetable Salad

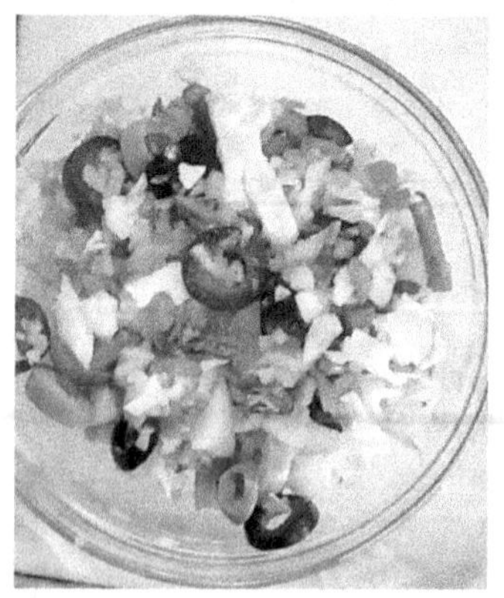

*I like to use my electric chopper for this recipe. A tip: don't combine vegetables when chopping. Chop each vegetable separately; chop all of your radish, remove and then chop your celery, remove and then chop your next vegetable…. And so on.*

Comments:……………………………………………

…………………………………………………………………………

…………………………………………………………………………

…………………………………………………………………………

The ingredients for the Cold Chopped Vegetable Salad can be whatever you like and have on hand. Here are some suggestions:

- Cabbage
- Asparagus
- Carrot
- Radish
- Yellow summer Squash
- Zucchini
- Celery
- jicama
- Riced cauliflower
- Scallions
- Olives (choose a variety)
- Fennel
- Cucumber

I like to toss my chopped salad in oil and vinegar. My preference is Balsamic Vinegar.

- 2 T. oil
- 1 T. balsamic vinegar
- Salt and pepper

# Recipe 24: Cold Cucumber Soup

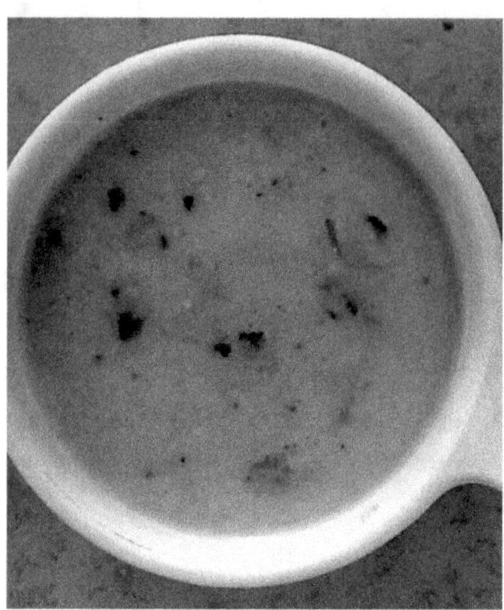

Ingredients

- 1 medium peeled cucumber
- 1 small ripe avocado, or ½ large avocado
- 1 T. oil
- 2 T. lime or lemon juice
- ½ cup cold water (approximately)
- 1/2 teaspoon salt (or more to taste)
- Pinch of black pepper

INSTRUCTIONS:

Blend all ingredients in your blender until smooth. Taste and adjust salt and lemon juice if needed to your taste. Best when allowed to then chill in the refrigerator for one full hour.

A delicious refreshing and hydrating soup!

This is delicious when you stir in a spoonful (or more) of the cucumber salsa (recipe 32) for a textured soup!

# Recipe 25: Cold Plate

This of course can have many substitutions.

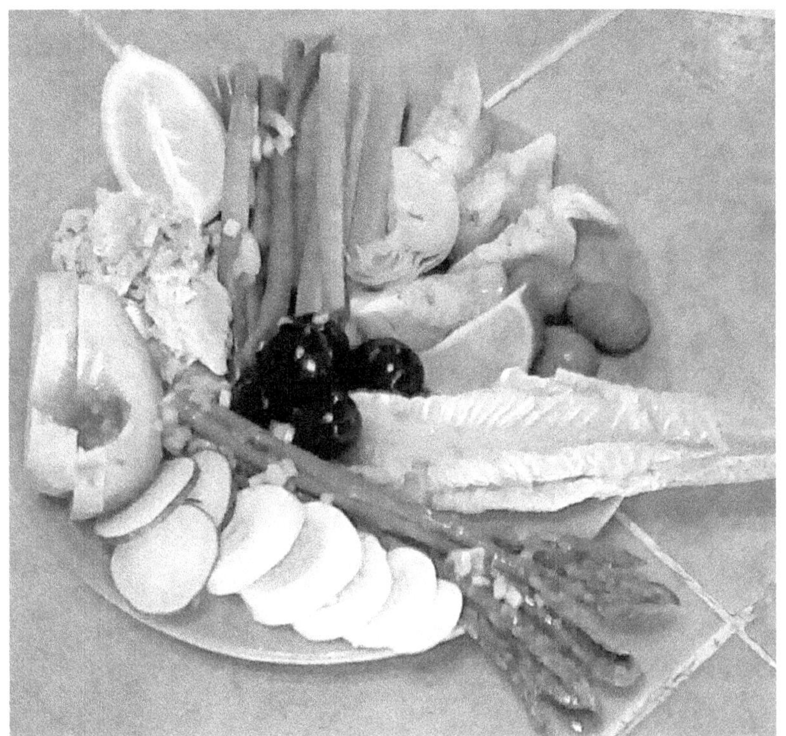

INGREDIENTS:

- Salmon, Tuna, or Cooked Chicken
- Boiled eggs
- Avocado
- Asparagus
- Romaine Hearts
- Radishes
- Artichokes
- Olives
- Carrots
- Green Beans
- Dressing of choice

# Recipe 26: Cold Vegetable Pizza

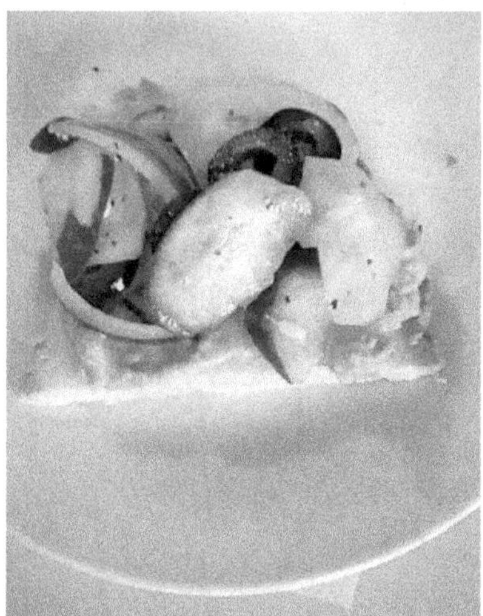

Pizza crust recipe 54, cooled or at least room temperature. Always a hit at a potluck!

Cold Vegetable Pizza Sauce:

- 1 Avocado
- ½ cup chopped peeled cucumber
- 1 T oil
- 1 t. apple cider vinegar
- Salt and pepper
- 1 t. Italian seasoning

Place all above ingredients for the sauce in a chopper or blender until smooth. Spread onto low carb Pizza Crust. Top with Salad. Can be refrigerated several days even with the toppings. *Best when chilled, with toppings, at least one hour.*

**Top it off** with Salad Vegetables: pictured is shaved cucumber, red onion and black olives tossed in oil, vinegar and Italian seasonings. But use whatever you like or have on hand. Sometimes I like to toss broccoli, shredded carrots, and chopped lettuce with my favorite dressing and put that on top!

# Recipe 27: Cream of Broccoli Soup

- 1 bunch fresh broccoli broken down into florets and include the tender part of the stalk
- 2 cups chicken broth
- 2 T. oil
- ½ t. apple cider vinegar
- 1 t. lemon juice
- Salt and pepper (lemon pepper is a great choice in this dish)

Instructions

1. Boil or steam your broccoli until tender. Drain but reserve the liquid.
2. Allow broccoli to cool.
3. Place all ingredients into your blender. Blend until smooth.
4. Add more broth if needed.
5. If you use all of your broth and find you need more liquid you can use the water from boiling the broccoli if you saved it.
6. Once you have the soup to the consistency you like transfer to a saucepan on the stove over medium heat.
7. Heat through. Best if allowed to simmer about 15 minutes or so.

The beauty of recipes like this one is that if you have someone who prefers cheese they can add it at the table.

# Recipe 28: Cream of Zucchini Soup

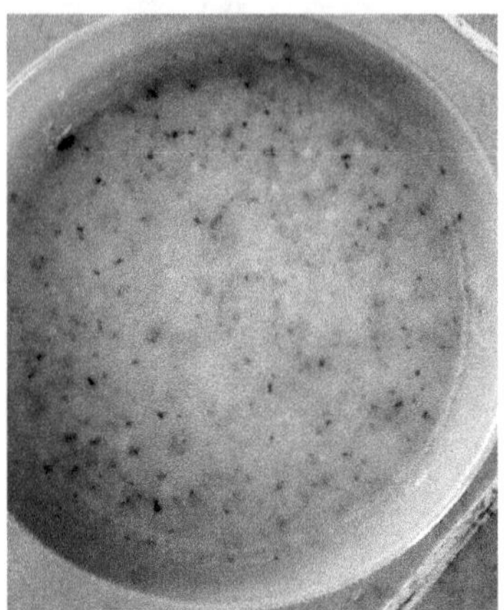

INGREDIENTS:

- 1 T. real unsalted butter
- 1 T. oil
- 2 cloves minced garlic
- 1 cup chicken broth
- Salt
- Lemon Pepper
- 1-2 Small to medium zucchini, cut into chunks

INSTRUCTIONS:

1. Sauté the garlic in the butter and oil in a saucepan until garlic is just tender and slightly brown. Remove the garlic from the saucepan.
2. Add the zucchini and broth, salt and lemon pepper to saucepan. Cover.
3. Boil until the zucchini is tender. About ten minutes.
4. Transfer to a bowl to allow time to cool down. About 30 minutes.
5. Add to your blender and blend until smooth.
6. Return to the saucepan with the garlic you set aside earlier and heat through.

# Recipe 29: Creamy Italian Dressing

- 1 cup mayo or try a ripe avocado and just ¼ cup may
- ¼ cup minced onion
- 2 T red wine vinegar
- 1 tsp Stevia
- 1 T Italian seasoning
- ¼ tsp garlic powder
- ¼ tsp salt
- 1/8 tsp black pepper
- 1 ounce oil

Blend all ingredients together. Chill at least one hour.

Comments:……………………………………………

………………………………………………………………………………………………………

………………………………………………………………………………………………………

………………………………………………………………………………………………………

# Recipe 30: Cucumber Salad

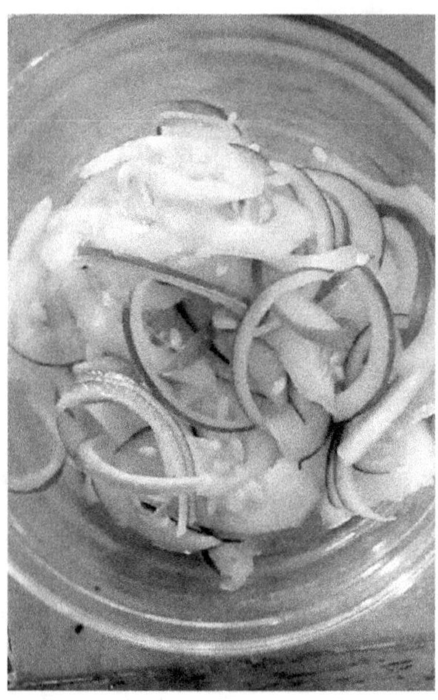

INGREDIENTS:

- 1 cup shaved Cucumbers (I like to use the side slicer on my grater)
- ½ cup sliced white or purple onions
- Sliced red radishes and cilantro (optional)

Basic dressing: 3 T. oil, 1 T. apple cider vinegar, salt and pepper OR you can use the Asian Dressing, Recipe 02

Mix dressing and vegetables. Chill at least one hour before serving.

# Recipe 31: Cucumber Salad Dressing

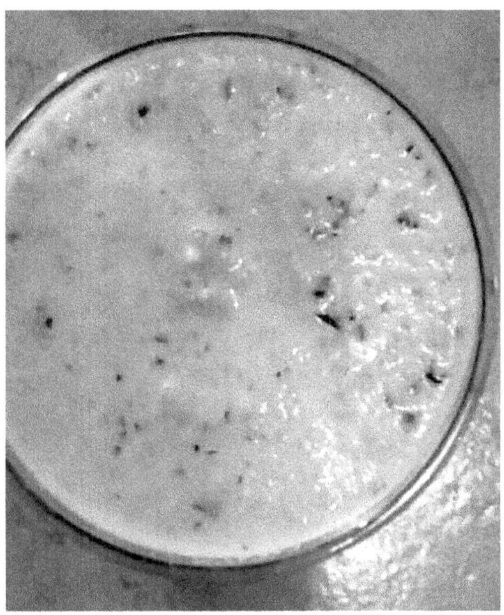

INGREDIENTS:

- ½ cucumber peeled and chopped. About one cup after chopping.
- ¼ cup oil
- 1 T. Apple cider vinegar
- ¼ t. salt and ¼ t. pepper

Blend all in blender. Keep in a glass jar in the refrigerator. Makes about ½ cup.

# Recipe 32: Cucumber Salsa

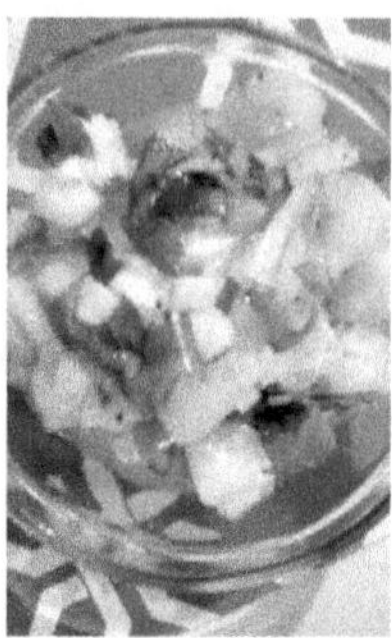

This is tomato free! This is not going to taste like a tomato salsa, but it does taste refreshing and delicious! The apple cider vinegar is absolutely necessary to this recipe. You can also replace the cucumber with watermelon!

- 1 cucumber, peeled and diced
- 1 T. white onion, diced
- ¾ cup chopped fresh cilantro
- 3-4 T. Oil
- 2 T. Lime juice
- 1 t. apple cider vinegar
- Salt and Pepper

Combine all ingredients. Best when allowed to chill at least one full hour before serving. This is very good stirred into the Cold Cucumber Soup Recipe 24. Also a nice accompaniment to fish and chicken dishes, or, mixed into salads or used as a dip!

Optional substitutions: use scallions instead of onions. Use purple onions for some color! Add some minced garlic cloves if you like garlic.

Anytime you slice a cucumber, be sure to taste a slice before adding to your recipe or serving. If it taste bitter, cover your remaining peeled cucumber with fresh water and refrigerate for about an hour. This should help to eliminate that bitter taste.

# Recipe 33: Deviled Eggs

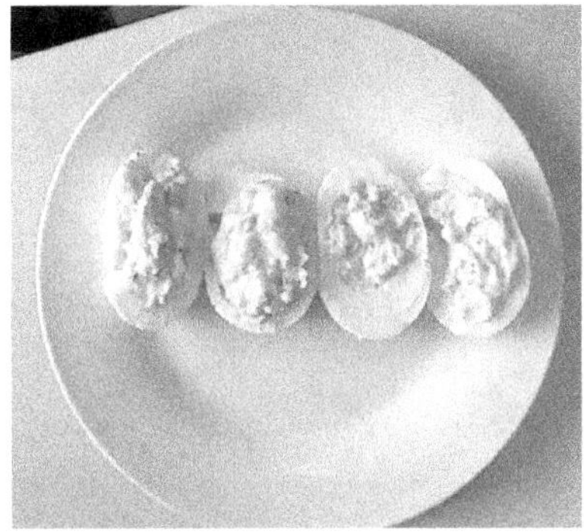

"Hard-cooked eggs are stuffed with a creamy blend of mayonnaise, Dijon mustard and rice wine vinegar. Fresh dill and garlic powder add a delightful flavor."

INGREDIENTS:

- 2 hard-cooked eggs, halved
- 2 Tbsp mayonnaise
- ½ teaspoon rice wine vinegar (just shy of ½ tsp)
- teaspoon dijon mustard
- garlic powder: a couple of quick shakes
- 1/8 teaspoon salt and pepper
- ½ teaspoon chopped scallions thinly sliced

Some tips before you start:
Mix the egg yolks with the other ingredients while still warm for a creamier deviled egg filling.
Boiled Egg Method: place eggs in cold water in your saucepan. Bring to a boil which takes approximately 10 minutes. As soon as the water is at a full boil remove saucepan from heat and cover tightly. Leave the eggs to sit for 11 minutes before draining and peeling. During that time get all of your other ingredients ready to go.

**INSTRUCTIONS:**

Scoop egg yolks into a bowl and set egg whites aside. Mash warm yolks, mayo, vinegar, Dijon mustard, garlic powder, salt, and pepper. Spoon yolk mixture into egg whites. Garnish with minced scallion greens. Refrigerate until ready to serve. Best when refrigerated for at least one full hour before serving.

# Recipe 34: Egg Salad

INGREDIENTS:

- 2 Boiled eggs (mix while the yolks are still warm)
- 3 T. mayo
- 1 t. Dijon mustard
- 2 T. diced celery
- 1/8 t celery seed
- Salt and pepper

Place eggs in cold water completely submerged. Bring to a full boil. Remove from heat. Cover. Wait 15 minutes. Peel, chop eggs coarsely, add to mixture of: mayo, mustard, celery, and seasonings.

Egg salad makes a nice sandwich for breakfast, lunch, or supper. You can also ditch the bread and instead use the egg salad as a dip with your Sunflower Seed Crackers Recipe 65, or in a healthy, low carb tortilla for a take-on-the-go wrap. I must admit that my favorite thing to do with egg salad is to place it on top a nice lettuce salad!

Comments:……………………………………………………

………………………………………………………………………………………

………………………………………………………………………………………

………………………………………………………………………………………

# Recipe 35: Fried Broccoli

INGREDIENTS

- 3 ounces oil
- 1 lb fresh broccoli
- 1 T minced garlic
- Salt and Lemon pepper
- 4 T. water

INSTRUCTIONS

1. Toss broccoli in oil, garlic, salt, and lemon pepper.
2. Transfer to heated skillet on medium heat.
3. Add water and cook broccoli, stirring occasionally, until tender!

Comments:……………………………………………

………………………………………………………………………………………

………………………………………………………………………………………

………………………………………………………………………………………

Recipe 35: Fried Broccoli

# Recipe 36: Green Bean Salad

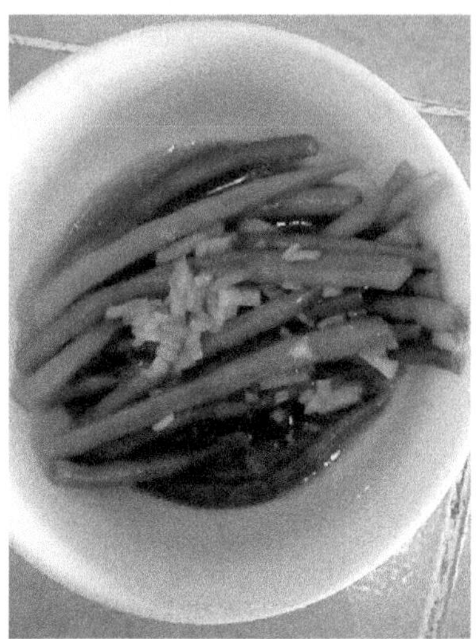

INGREDIENTS:

- ½ pound fresh green beans, ends trimmed
- Asian Dressing, Recipe 02
- 4 Tablespoons minced onion
- 2 large garlic cloves, minced

Comments:……………………………………………

……………………………………………………………………………

……………………………………………………………………………

……………………………………………………………………………

INSTRUCTIONS:

1. I like to make the dressing first and set aside so the flavors can marry.
2. Make the Asian Dressing, Recipe 02. Add the minced onion and garlic to your prepared dressing. Set aside.
3. Bring a large pot of water to a boil. Add 1 teaspoon salt.
4. Cook green beans until tender, 15 minutes.
5. While they cook, prepare a large bowl with an ice water bath. Immediately drain the beans into a colander (or scoop them out with a slotted spoon) and place the drained beans in the ice water for a few minutes to stop the cooking. This will keep them bright green and perfectly tender.
6. Drain the beans and pat them dry.

Pour dressing mixture over the green beans and toss to coat. Cover the bowl and chill for at least an hour or up to 3 hours before ready to serve.
Serve chilled or at room temperature.
NOTES:
The desired tenderness of the green beans is a personal preference so check them often

Comments:……………………………………………

………………………………………………………………………………………

………………………………………………………………………………………

………………………………………………………………………………………

# Recipe 37: Green Beans, poached

- 1 lb fresh green beans, washed and trimmed
- 2 cups chicken broth
- 2 garlic cloves, minced
- 2 T oil
- Salt and Pepper

Instructions

1. Place broth and beans in skillet or saucepan with lid.
2. Poach beans in chicken broth and garlic for about 15 minutes. Should be tender but not mushy.
3. Remove beans from broth to a large bowl. Toss with oil, salt and pepper.

Comments:…………………………………………

……………………………………………………………………

……………………………………………………………………

……………………………………………………………………

Recipe 37: Green Beans, poached

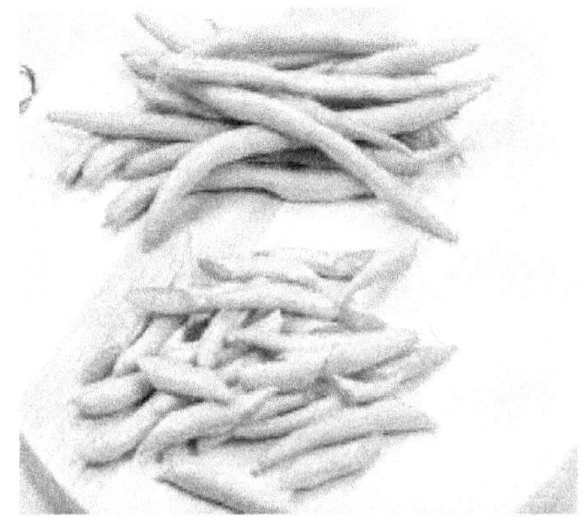

Green Beans are very healthy!

According to organicfacts.net the fiber content of green beans is very high. Green beans are a good source for vitamin A, C, K, B6, folic acid, calcium, silicon, iron, manganese, potassium, and copper.

# Recipe 38: Ground Turkey Lettuce Cups

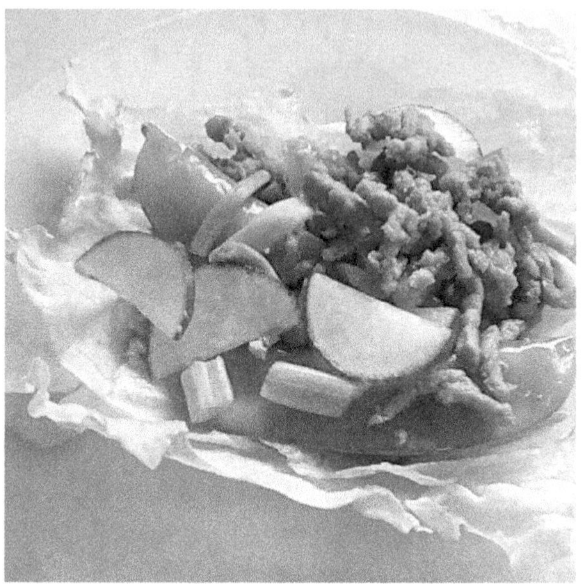

Ingredients:

- ½ lb ground ground Turkey (Styrofoam)
- 2 T. oil
- Asian Dressing (recipe 02)
- ….with minced onions and garlic

Toppings
- ¼ cup sliced scallions
- ¼ cup sliced radishes
- ¼ cup sliced cucumbers
- ¼ cup shredded carrots

Fresh lettuce of your choice that will form a nice cup. It helps to layer two or three leaves for stability.

1. Make the Asian Dressing, Recipe 02 and add to it a tablespoon minced onion and a teaspoon of minced garlic. Set aside.

2. Brown the ground turkey in a skillet with oil. When halfway browned, add ½ the Asian Dressing, setting some aside to use as a topping at the table.
3. Allow the turkey to simmer, and finish cooking, in the Asian Dressing, for about 10-15 minutes.
4. While the turkey is cooking get your lettuce cups ready on a plate.


Spoon the finished turkey into each lettuce cup and top with your choice of fresh thinly sliced red onion, cucumber, radishes, scallions, shredded carrots or even a light slaw.
Drizzle with a bit more Asian Dressing.
This dish pairs well with fried broccoli stir fry, recipe 35 or even the Roasted Cauliflower Steaks, Recipe 55.


Comments:…………………………………………

……………………………………………………………………………

……………………………………………………………………………

……………………………………………………………………………

# Recipe 39: Guacamole Dip

- 2 ripe avocados
- 1/8 cup onion, finely chopped
- 1/8 cup Chopped Cilantro
- Lime Juice (to taste) Start with a teaspoon
- 1 T. oil
- Salt to taste, and black pepper
- 1/4 cup cucumber, diced

I like to use my electric food chopper for this one.
Just place all of your ingredients in the chopper and pulse until blended.

# Recipe 40: Horseradish Mayo

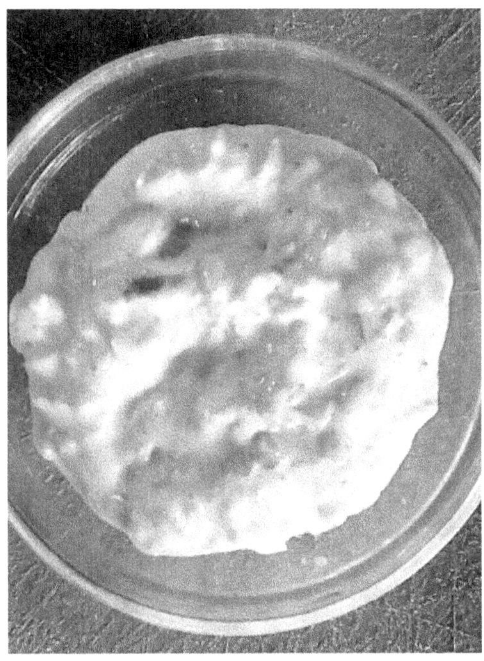

**INGREDIENTS:**

¼ cup rustic chopped onion
1 T. Dill Relish
¾ cup mayonnaise
1 t. prepared horseradish
2 t. drained capers
2 t. Dijon mustard
1 celery stalk chopped. About ½ cup

INSTRUCTIONS:

Blend all ingredients in your chopper or blender until somewhat smooth. Taste and then add salt (or not) to suit your taste. Can chill in refrigerator in glass jar for up to 7 days.

This is a great sandwich spread, dip, or sauce for grilled romaine, salad dressing for a salad, use in place of tartar sauce for fish.

# Recipe 41: Italian Dressing

INGREDIENTS ·


- 1 garlic clove, minced
- 1 t.  minced onion
- ¼  tsp granulated Stevia
- ½ t. Italian seasoning
- Pinch of black pepper and pinch of salt
- 1/3 cup Oil
- ¼ cup Red wine Vinegar
- ½ t. Apple Cider Vinegar

INSTRUCTIONS


1. In a glass jar combine all ingredients. Cover with tight lid. Shake well to combine.

2. Best after refrigerated at least one hour.


Comments:……………………………………………

………………………………………………………………………………

………………………………………………………………………………

………………………………………………………………………………

# Recipe 42: Italian Sausage

- 1/2 lb ground pork
- 2 T. Italian Seasoning
- 1/2 tsp garlic powder
- 1/2 tsp onion powder
- 1/2 tsp thyme
- 1/2 tsp sea salt
- 1/2 tsp coarsely-ground black pepper

## Instructions:

1. Mix meat with dried spices
2. Crumble and brown in large greased skillet or form into patties or meatballs. Cook as appropriate to your recipe or meal plans. Also great on Pizza Crust Recipe 54.


Comments:…………………………………………………

………………………………………………………………………………………………

………………………………………………………………………………………………

………………………………………………………………………………………………

## Recipe 43: Kraut Sauté

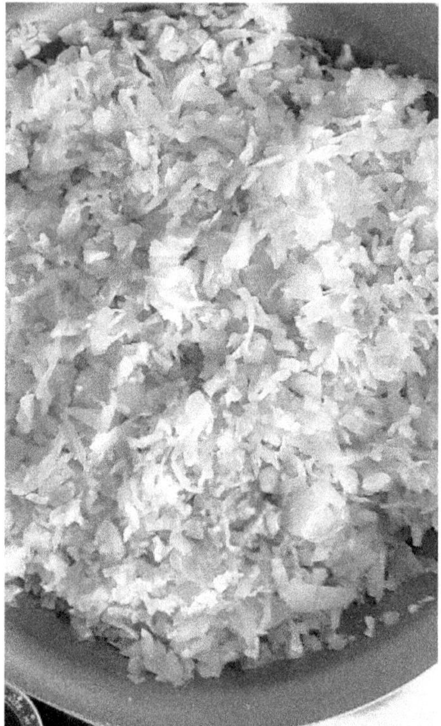

Pictured here without the pork

Ingredients:

- 1 lb ground pork
- ½ cup diced onion
- ½  cup diced carrot
- 1 cup diced celery
- 1 (14oz) can kraut (the only ingredients should be cabbage, water and salt)
- 2 T oil
- 2 T. ground Sage
- 1 T. thyme

You can dice the vegetables in less than 5 minutes if you use a chopper!

## Instructions:

Combine all ingredients in a skillet on medium to high heat. Spread evenly and sort of press into the pan.

Leave for about 10 minutes allowing any liquid to cook out and a bit of browning to occur on the bottom. Then, stir until heated through.

Make this a great entrée by adding ground pork and season with sage and/or thyme. Or, makes a great side dish with a hamburger patty steak: mix fresh (never been frozen) hamburger with salt and pepper and 1 T oil. Form patties and fry like a hamburger. Plate like a steak.

## Recipe 44: Lemon Herb Salmon

- 2 salmon filets
- 2 T. oil
- 1 T. brown sugar (about 8 carbs spread out over dish = about 4 carbs per serving)
- 1 T. lemon juice
- 1 T. Dijon mustard
- 1 garlic clove, minced
- 1 t. oregano
- Salt and pepper

1. Preheat your oven to 400 degrees.
2. In a bowl, combine sugar, mustard lemon juice, garlic, oregano, oil, salt and pepper. Set aside.
3. Line baking sheet with foil.
4. Toss the salmon with oil and seasonings/juice.
5. Close up foil.
6. Bake about 18 minutes.


Comments:………………………………………

………………………………………………………………………………

………………………………………………………………………………

……………………………………Paula C. Henderson…………………………

## Recipe 46: Lemon Vinaigrette

1 T. fresh squeezed lemon juice
¼ t. Dijon mustard
½ t. white sugar (2 carbs)
1 T. Oil
Salt and pepper to taste

Combine all ingredients in a glass jar. Cover and shake well. This is a nice choice to use with the Asparagus Salad Recipe 04

Comments:………………………………………………

……………………………………………………………………………………………

……………………………………………………………………………………………

……………………………………………………………………………………………

# Recipe 47: Mashed Cauliflower

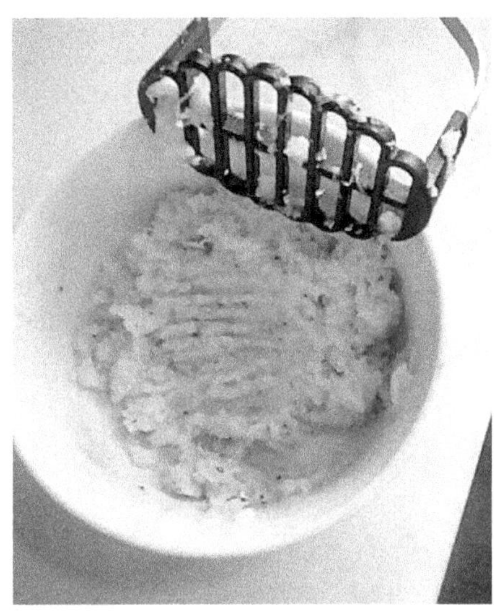

**Ingredients**

- 2 T extra virgin olive oil or real, unsalted butter
- dash of salt and dash of pepper to taste
- One head medium cauliflower

INSTRUCTIONS

1. Chop cauliflower. Boil until very tender (about 15 to 20 minutes)
2. Drain well. I like to use my hand held masher and mash the cauliflower while in the strainer to get as much of the liquid out as I can.
3. Scoop the cauliflower into your serving bowl and add oil or butter, salt and pepper.
4. Mash again if you feel you need to and then using a spoon, combine very well.
5. You should not feel the need to add liquid, but if you do you can add water, chicken broth, or liquid you boiled the cauliflower in. Start with just a couple tablespoons if any at all.

Make extra and use to make Cauliflower "potato" pancakes Recipe 13, for another meal!

This Mashed Cauliflower recipe is also the topping for Shepard's Pie Recipe 64

# Recipe 48: Meatballs

*Be sure to use ground beef that has never been frozen and is at least 80% lean.*

**INGREDIENTS:**

1 pound ground hamburger
2 T Oil
4 Tbsp Italian Seasoning or if you want a more basic taste profile replace with thyme
1 Tablespoon minced onion
1 Tbsp minced celery
1 Tbsp garlic powder (not salt)
1 tsp salt
1 tsp pepper
½ cup water or broth

**INSTRUCTIONS:**

Mix all ingredients together and form golf ball size balls.

Brown lightly on all sides in medium skillet. Add ½ cup water to skillet. Using a spatula, scrape the bottom of the skillet. Cover with a lid and let simmer about 5 minutes. May need to turn your burner down slightly. Remove the lid and return the burner to medium heat. Cook on all sides until a more golden brown. Always be sure to make an extra to check for doneness and seasonings.

Comments:…………………………………………………

…………………………………………………………………………

…………………………………………………………………………

…………………………………………………………………………

# Recipe 49: Meatloaf

*Be sure to use ground beef that has never been frozen and is at least 80% lean.*

**INGREDIENTS:**

- 1 lb 80% or leaner Ground Beef in the Styrofoam tray. Not the tube.
- 2 T's oil
- 4 T Italian Seasoning
- 1/3 cup minced onion
- 1/3 cup minced celery
- ½ tsp salt and ½ tsp pepper

Combine all ingredients in a glass bowl. Form into a meatloaf shape.

Bake at 375 degrees for 30 minutes per pound.

Comments:……………………………………………

……………………………………………………………………………………………

……………………………………………………………………………………………

……………………………………………………………………………………………

# Recipe 50: Mushroom Gravy

**INGREDIENTS**:

- 8 ounce package sliced mushrooms (cremini or ports are highly suggested)
- 1/8 cup oil
- ½ t. garlic powder or minced garlic
- Salt and pepper
- 2 T. Real, Unsalted Butter
- 1 cup White Wine or Vermouth (or broth of choice)
- 1 T. lemon juice
- Cornstarch

**Instructions**:

1. Toss the sliced mushrooms with oil, salt, pepper and garlic.
2. Sauté in hot skillet until the mushrooms start to look toasted.
3. Sprinkle the mushrooms very lightly with cornstarch.
4. Add butter and wine. Stirring well. Sauce should thicken. Simmer about 3-5 minutes stirring occasionally.
5. Remove from heat. Toss with cilantro or parsley and the lemon juice.

If you feel the sauce is too thin, remove some sauce to a small bowl and make a slurry using a tablespoon of cornstarch. Bring remaining sauce back to a low simmer on the stove and stir in the slurry until well blended.

# Recipe 51: Olive Salad

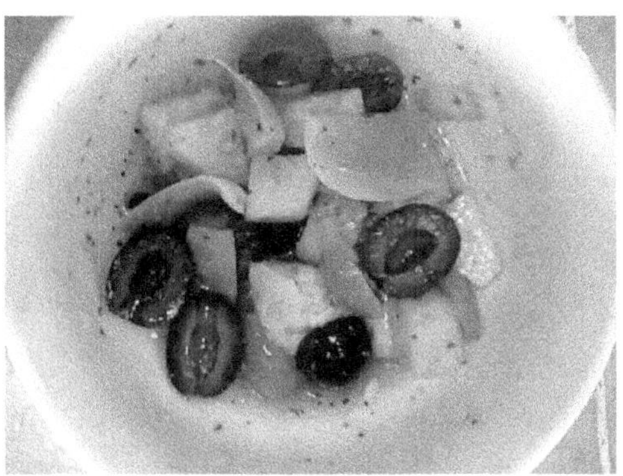

**INGREDIENTS**:

- 4 small artichoke hearts
- ½ cup quartered cucumber: chop into bite size pieces
- 8 large black olives cut in half
- 8 Kalamata olives
- 1 T. oil
- 1 t. Balsamic Vinegar
- Salt and pepper
- 1 garlic cloves, minced

Toss all ingredients together and chill in glass container with lid.

Excellent tossed with leftover grilled/roasted vegetables or even a lettuce salad!

Comments:………………………………………………

………………………………………………………………………………

………………………………………………………………………………

# Recipe 52: Pesto (dairy free and nut free)

**INGREDIENTS**:

2 cups fresh spinach leaves
1 Tbsp garlic cloves - minced
1 Tbsp lemon juice
¼ tsp salt
¼ cup olive oil
2 large Minced garlic cloves

Instructions:
Place all ingredients in a food processor and pulse until rustic-ly mixed and chopped.

# Recipe 53: Pillowed Spinach

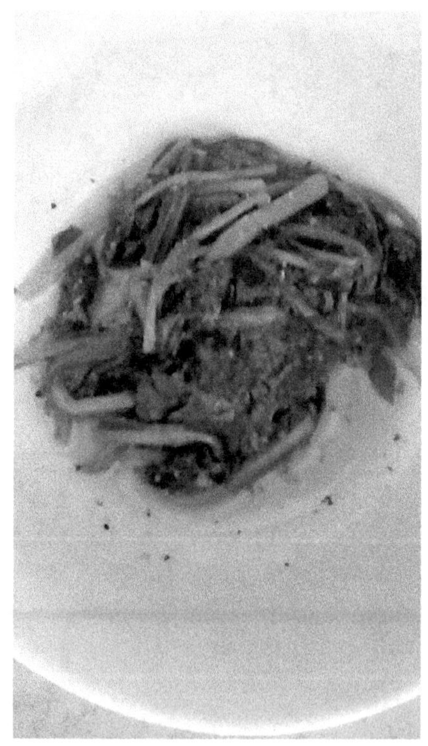

INGREDIENTS:

- 1 bunch of fresh spinach
- 2-4 T. Oil
- 1 T. Italian seasoning
- 1 t. garlic powder
- Salt and pepper
- 2-4 T. water

INSTRUCTIONS:

1. Combine oil and seasonings in a cold skillet.
2. Heat skillet over medium to high heat.
3. Spread spinach evenly over the top of the broth. Do Not Stir.
4. Drizzle water over top of spinach. Do NOT stir.
5. Cover with a lid and simmer for about 3 minutes. Remove from heat.
6. Spinach should be soft. Taste spinach and see if texture is to your liking. Should be tender, soft and pillow-y.
7. Gently fold the spinach into the oil and seasonings.
8. Use a slotted spoon and remove the spinach.
9. This technique can be used with any other dish you want to pair spinach with: chicken, fish, beef, pork, sautéed mushrooms, and other vegetables. Just add your fresh spinach to top of the contents in your skillet during the last 5 minutes of cooking. Do not stir. If you have broth on the bottom just lay the spinach on top and cover with a lid for about 3 minutes.

Set your grilled or baked chicken breasts, steak or pork chop right on top!


Comments:………………………………………………

……………………………………………………………………………………………

……………………………………………………………………………………………

……………………………………………………………………………………………

# Recipe 54: Pizza Crust (easy!)

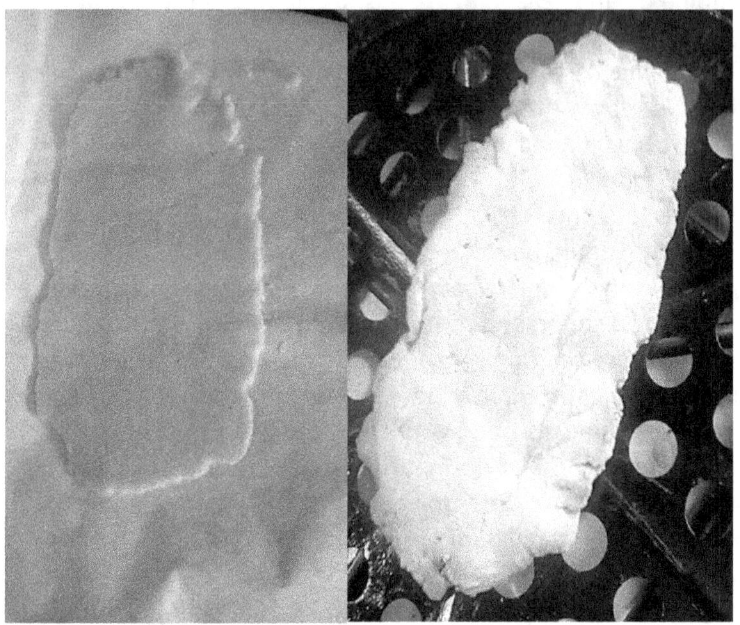

**INGREDIENTS:**

- ½ cup Almond flour
- 1 small egg or ½ of a whisked large egg
- ¼  t. xanthan gum
- 1 t. melted real unsalted butter (if substituting use something you have to melt)

You will also need parchment paper, pizza pan with holes, and nonstick cooking spray.

**INSTRUCTIONS:**

1. Preheat oven to 350 degrees.
2. Combine all ingredients in a bowl. Dough will be wet.
3. Form a ball using a spoon and let rest at least 10 minutes.
4. After sitting the ball should be much drier than before.
5. Work the dough for a couple minutes.

6. Place the dough between two pieces of parchment paper and roll out to about ¼" thin.
7. I generally make a rectangle, using a rolling pin and it rolls to about 8 inches long and 3-4 inches wide.
8. Spray your pizza pan with nonstick cooking spray.
9. Remove the top paper from the dough and then, lifting the parchment paper with the dough on it,  turn the dough over onto the pizza pan.

10. Bake at 350 degrees in a preheated oven until starting to turn a golden brown. About 15 minutes.
11. Remove and let cool slightly (about 10 minutes) before adding your favorite toppings.

If making traditional hot pizza:

Add your favorite pizza toppings (after the initial cooking time above) and then return to the oven (350) until toppings have heated through. Watch the crust so as to not over brown or burn. Use the broiler instead if needed. About another 10 minutes when put back into the oven.

*If using this for the Cold Vegetable Pizza: this only needs baked the one time (350 for 15 minutes). Allow to cool before topping. Will keep in frig well until ready to eat. I generally go ahead and put my toppings on if I will be eating within the next 24 hours. Best when chilled, with toppings, at least one hour.*

Comments:……………………………………………

………………………………………………………………………………………

………………………………………………………………………………………

………………………………………………………………………………………

# Recipe 55: Roasted Cabbage Steaks

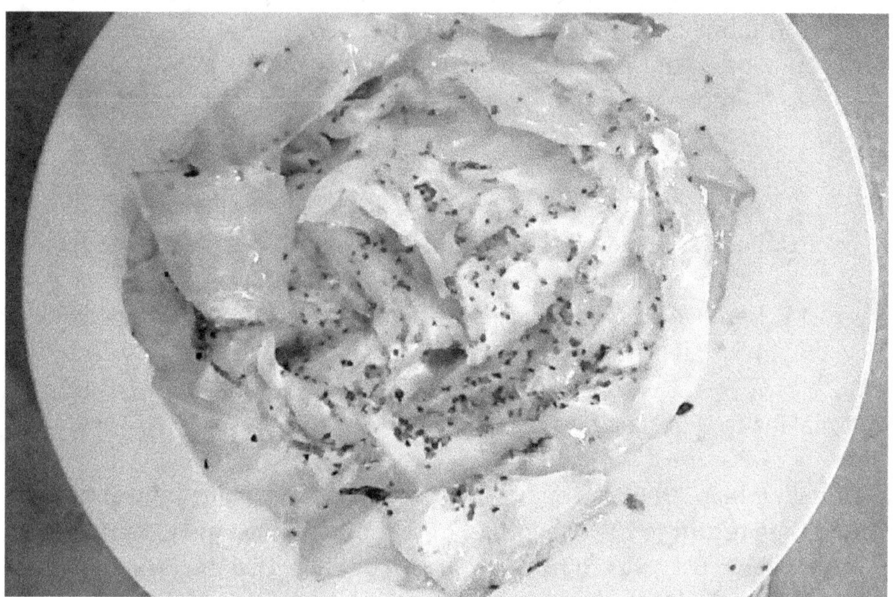

**INGREDIENTS**

- Cabbage slices
- Oil
- Salt
- Lemon pepper

Slice cabbage into steaks. Drizzle with oil. Salt and pepper.
Bake in a preheated 400 degrees, 25-30 minutes or until tender.

# Recipe 56: Roasted Chicken

**INGREDIENTS**:

- 6 lb Hen  (completely thawed! set out on the counter for 30 minutes before preparing to bake)
- Oil
- Salt and Pepper (lemon pepper is nice too)

**INSTRUCTIONS**:

1. Clear out the cavity. You can place some seasonings inside the cavity if you wish. Some suggestions would be:
2. Garlic and Lemon wedge
3. Rosemary and Thyme with lemon wedge
4. Cumin, sage and lemon wedge
5. Preheat oven to 375 degrees.
6. Rub the entire hen with oil, then rub salt and pepper into the skin.
7. Place on baking sheet or roasting pan.
8. Place into a preheated oven with a loose bit of aluminum foil on top. The hen should be breasts side up.
9. Bake a 3 lb hen for an hour and a half. Do not baste. Do not open the oven door until the last half hour in order to remove the foil. Turn the oven up to 425 degrees the last 15 minutes only.
10. Remove from oven. Always allow the hen to set at least 30 minutes before slicing.

Tips: Generally speaking: Allow 20 minutes per pound plus 15 more minutes at the end on higher heat or using the broil for about 5 to brown the top. All ovens are different so you will need to watch this the first time you cook it and adjust accordingly to suit your oven.

# Recipe 57: Roasted Vegetables

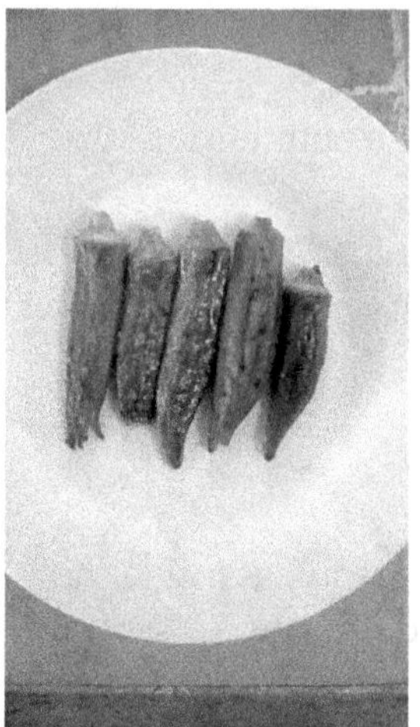

This is a picture of blistered okra. I use frozen okra most of the year as it is difficult to find fresh in the produce department year round. Just prepare it as instructed below straight out of the freezer.

Roasting almost any vegetable couldn't be easier or healthier and so tasty you'll wonder why you haven't been doing it all along! Enjoy as a side dish, your main dish, Hot or Cold! Tossed as a roasted vegetable salad, or even make a sandwich. Prepare on your grill or in your oven. Just give them a try!

Sometimes I use just one vegetable; like roasted Brussels sprouts or whole okra. Other times, I like to roast 2-4 vegetables together. There really are no rules as to which vegetables you might like so try what sounds good to you. Here are some suggestions though.

- Fresh quartered onions
- Fresh zucchini (sliced) (best when done lengthwise on a grill)
- Fresh Brussels Sprouts (always cut in half)
- Fresh cauliflower, cut florets in half to expose the inside
- Whole frozen okra (leave as is)
- Oil

## INSTRUCTIONS

1. Slice and chop vegetables how you like. Sometimes for presentation but no smaller than a large bite size.
2. Toss with Salt, Pepper, and enough oil to coat. Use a large glass or stainless steel bowl to give you room for tossing.
3. Spread onto a baking sheet. Try not to crowd them too much.
4. Bake in a preheated oven at 450 degrees for about 15 minutes or until golden brown and tender. With some, you might like to hit them with the broiler to brown and blister the tops!

Try using any leftover roasted vegetables in a cold salad, tossed with some balsamic vinegar.

# Recipe 58: Salsa Verde

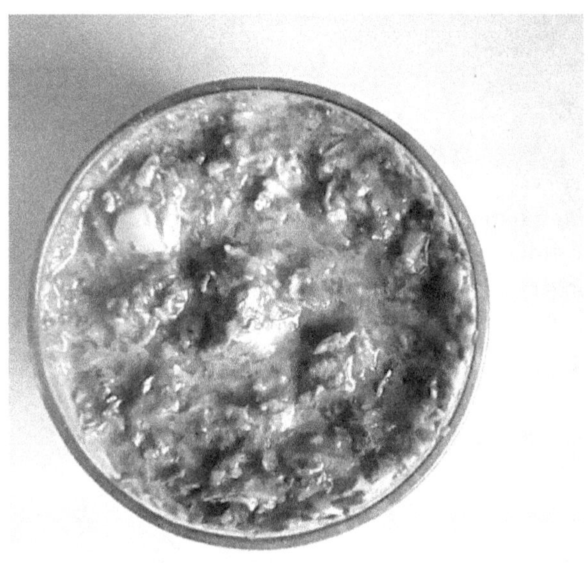

**INGREDIENTS**

1 cup rough chopped Cilantro
1 T. rough chopped onion
4 T. Oil
1 T. ACV (apple cider vinegar)
¼ t. Salt
¼ t. pepper

Place all in a *chopper. Pulse until mixed well. A rustic chop. Taste and adjust salt, pepper, and vinegar if necessary. Best after set on counter at room temperature for about an hour before serving. Saves in a glass jar in refrigerator for up to 4 days. Nice "relish" on meats, fish, vegetables, or toss in a salad.

# Recipe 59: Salisbury Steaks with Mushroom Gravy

*Be sure to use ground beef that has never been frozen and is at least 80% lean.*

## Steaks:

- 1 lb ground hamburger
- 1 large egg
- 2 garlic cloves, minced
- ¼ cup minced onion (either grate: this creates minced onion plus the juice, or use your chopper)
- ½ t. red wine vinegar
- 2 T. Dijon mustard
- 1 t. onion powder
- 2 T. oil for mixture and another 1 T. for skillet
- ½ t. salt
- ¼ t. black pepper

1. Combine all ingredients in a bowl. Form into Salisbury steak patties. Like mini meatloaf's about the thickness of a regular hamburger only oval.
2. Add a T. oil to skillet.
3. Brown steaks on both sides, about 3 minutes each side. Remove from the skillet. Your steaks will finish cooking inside when they are returned to the skillet later.

Comments:…………………………………………………

……………………………………………………………………………………

……………………………………………………………………………………

## Gravy:
1 (8) ounce pkg sliced mushrooms
1 T. minced onion
2 large garlic cloves, minced

# Recipe 45: Lemon and Olive Chicken

5 large green olives, 5 Kalamata olives, 5 black olives
1 T. lemon juice
2 ribs celery, chopped
4 garlic cloves
2 bay leaves
1 onion, chopped
1 bulb, fennel, cored and chopped
4 boneless chicken breast with the rib or thighs
¾ cup chicken broth
½ cup chopped fresh parsley
½ t. dried oregano
Salt and pepper to taste

Put all ingredients in your crock pot except: lemon juice, and bit of chopped parsley for garnish. Leave to cook all day on low, about 6-8 hours or on high, 4 hours.
Just before serving add the lemon juice and fresh chopped parsley.

Comments:…………………………………………

…………………………………………………………………………………………

…………………………………………………………………………………………

…………………………………………………………………………………………

2 T. unsalted butter or oil
1 t. Dijon mustard
1 t. rice vinegar
1 ½ cups Beef broth
½ cup water
2 T. cornstarch

1. Sauté the mushrooms in the skillet, scraping the bottom for renderings from the Salisbury steaks. After just a couple minutes, about 2 minutes, add the onion and garlic. Allow to cook over medium heat to soften the vegetables.

2. In small bowl combine: mustard, vinegar, and broth.

3. Add the 2 T. cornstarch to your vegetables in the skillet and stir around to coat.

4. Slowly add the liquid from your bowl to the skillet, stirring constantly. Broth should thicken to a nice brown gravy.
5. Add the meat steaks back into the skillet with the gravy. Turn over to coat both sides. Cover and allow to simmer on low about 10 minutes. Be sure you still have a bit of liquid on reserve in case it gets too thick. You can always add more beef broth or just a little water to thin it out if you need to.

Comments:………………………………………………

………………………………………………………………………………………

………………………………………………………………………………………

………………………………………………………………………………………

## Recipe 60: Salmon Patties

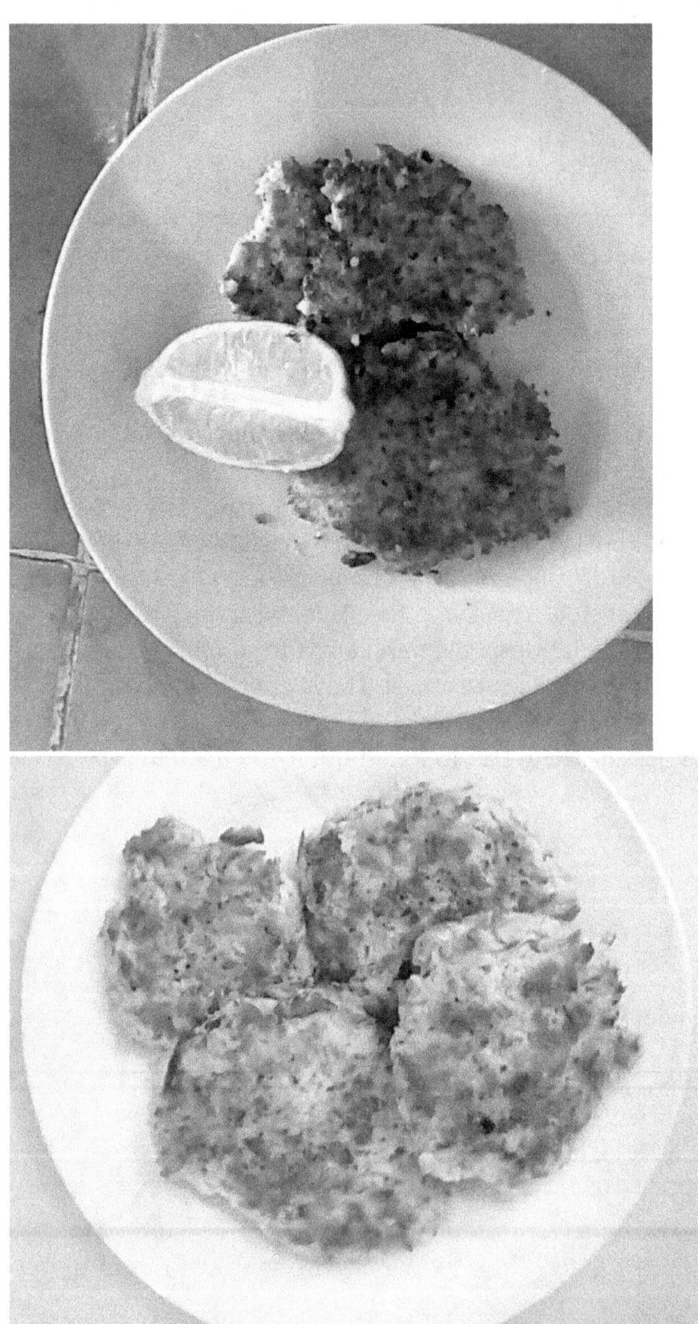

## INGREDIENTS

- *1 small egg
- 1/8 tsp garlic powder
- Lemon juice, I squeeze the juice from one quarter of a fresh lemon
- A pinch of salt
- ¼ t. celery seed or omit the salt and use celery salt instead
- ¼ t. thyme
- ¼ t. Lemon Pepper
- (1) 5 ounce  cans skinless boneless salmon (chicken or tuna)
- 3 T. oil

*I generally keep large eggs in the frig, and for this recipe I whisk one large egg in a small bowl, and then only use half per 5 ounce can of salmon, tuna or chicken. If using two 5 ounce cans I use the whole small egg. If using a 15 ounce can I use 2 large eggs.

## INSTRUCTIONS

1. Mix all ingredients together well. Press gently into a wire mesh strainer to remove excess liquid.
2. Heat oil in skillet over medium.
3. Using a spoon, spoon the mixture into skillet. Should make 2 medium patties.
4. Cook patties until both sides are a golden brown. About 4-5 minutes on each side.
5. DO NOT PRESS PATTIES WHILE COOKING.

# Recipe 61: Sautéed Mushrooms

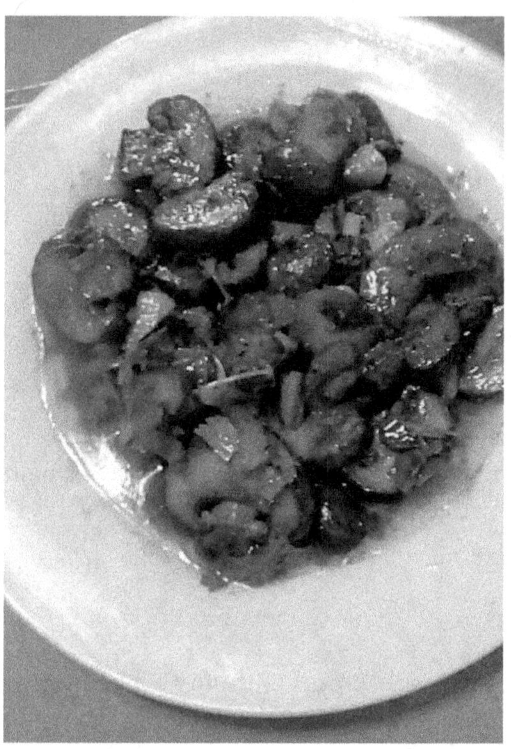

- 8 ounce package sliced mushrooms (cremini or ports are highly suggested)
- 1/8 cup oil
- ½ t. garlic powder or minced garlic
- Salt and pepper
- 1 T. Real, Unsalted Butter
- ¼ cup White Wine, Vermouth or chicken stock
- 1 T. lemon juice

## INSTRUCTIONS:

1. Toss the sliced mushrooms with oil, salt, pepper and garlic.
2. Sauté in hot skillet until the mushrooms start to look toasted.
3. Add butter and wine. Stirring well. Sauce should thicken. Simmer about 3-5 minutes stirring occasionally.
4. Remove from heat. Toss with cilantro or parsley and the lemon juice.
5. Some like just the mushrooms without additional sauce. If you like sauce, and your mushrooms seems to have plenty but you feel it is too thin, remove some sauce to a small bowl and make a slurry using a tablespoon of cornstarch. Bring remaining sauce back to a low simmer on the stove and stir in the slurry until well blended.

Comments:………………………………………….

………………………………………………………………………………………

………………………………………………………………………………………

………………………………………………………………………………………

# Recipe 62: Scallion Pancake

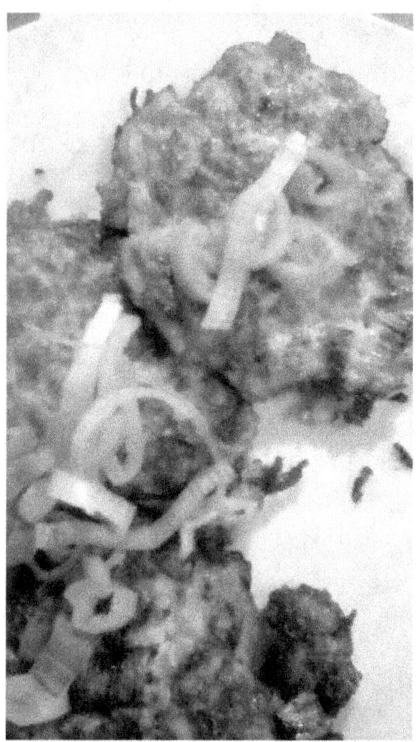

## INGREDIENTS

- 1½ cups mashed cauliflower
- One egg
- 2 scallions, sliced
- ½ teaspoon garlic powder
- Salt and pepper

INSTRUCTIONS:

1. Start with the mashed cauliflower Recipe 47, or with raw cauliflower:
2. Boil cauliflower until completely cooked and tender. Drain. Use a hand held masher to mash cauliflower well. Then, press cauliflower in a metal mesh strainer to get all of the water out you can.
3. Mix cauliflower with an egg and seasonings.
4. Fold in sliced scallions.
5. Heat a skillet with oil.
6. Fry these on medium heat about 7 minutes on the first side, and about 3-5 minutes on the second side.

Comments:...........................................

..............................................................................................

..............................................................................................

..............................................................................................

# Recipe 63: Seared Romaine

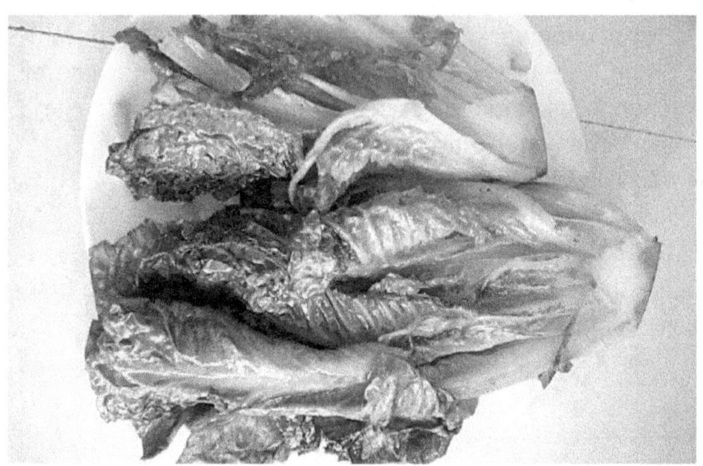

## INGREDIENTS

- Romaine hearts
- Oil
- Salt, pepper
- Balsamic

1. Cut the romaine hearts lengthwise.
2. Drizzle oil in skillet or grill pan.
3. Place romaine, inside flat side down onto skillet that should be on medium to high heat for searing.
4. Only takes a few moments.
5. Salt, pepper, and drizzle romaine hearts with balsamic vinegar or your favorite dressing.

# Recipe 64: Shepard's Pie

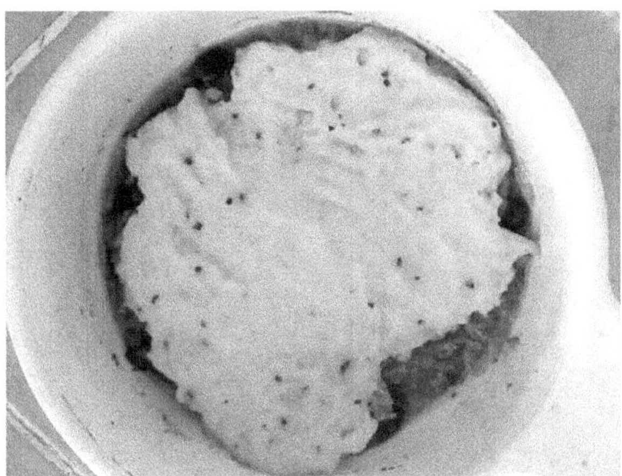

This is easy peasy! Combine 2 other recipes to make this one.

- Mashed Cauliflower, Recipe 47
- Vegetable Beef Soup, Recipe 74

1. Drain and retain, the liquid from the soup leaving just a bit with the meat and vegetables for moistness.

2. Spray your casserole dish with a nonstick cooking spray.
3. Add your drained Vegetable Beef Soup.

4. Combine your leftover mashed cauliflower with one large egg per one cup of cauliflower.
5. Top your casserole with the mashed cauliflower.

6. Use the liquid to drizzle over the top (optional) and offer cheese to top it off for those eating dairy.

Bake at 400 for about 20 minutes.

# Recipe 65: Sunflower Seed Crackers

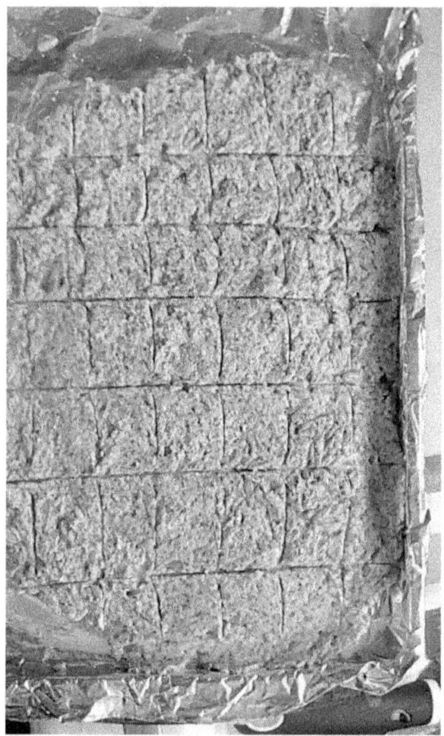

These crackers are the texture of a Triscuit. You can use whatever seasoning profile you favor. Here we are using rosemary but you could use garlic or onion powder instead if you prefer.

- ½ cup almond meal
- ½ cup ground flax seed meal
- ½ cup water
- 4 T.  shelled sunflower seeds
- ¼ tsp salt
- ½ t. dried rosemary

**INSTRUCTIONS**:

1. Mix the almond flour, flaxseed meal, water, sunflower seeds and seasonings. Stir well and set aside until water is absorbed and the dough holds together. About 5 minutes.
2. Preheat oven to 400 degrees
3. Turn dough onto the baking sheet (dough will be wet) that has been lined with parchment paper that has been sprayed with nonstick cooking spray. Lay another piece of parchment paper (also sprayed) on top of the dough. Press dough onto the prepared baking sheet.
4. Dough should be thin, like a cracker! Gently remove the parchment paper from the top.
5. Using a knife, score the dough as if you are making your crackers. Should make about 30 crackers.
6. Baked in PREHEATED 400 degree oven about 15-20 minutes.
7. Remove and allow to cool completely.

A note about making sure these crisp up! Be sure to bake them long enough. If you take them out too soon they will not crisp up. If once cooled, you find they are soft, you can put them back in the oven. The trick is getting them to start to turn a golden brown ( a sign of crisping) but not burning them. Every oven is so different. This is one of those recipes where you may take a couple of times to figure it out but once you do these are quite simply and quick to make.
If you successfully create about 30 crackers, each cracker will have approximately 1 carb. A traditional Triscuit has 3 carbs per cracker, compared to a saltine that has 7 carbs per cracker. Neither of those are gluten and soy free whereas this recipe is gluten free as well as soy free.

Comments:...............................................

...........................................................................................

...........................................................................................

...........................................................................................

# Recipe 66: Shrimp Scampi Carbonara

**INGREDIENTS**

¼ cup chopped bacon
1/4 cup avocado oil or mild olive oil
4 T. unsalted real butter or healthy oil
1 pounds shrimp, peeled and deveined
3 cloves garlic, minced
1 T. minced onion
4 tablespoons lemon juice (about 2 lemons, squeezed)
1/2 cup dry white wine or vermouth
1 1/2 tablespoons fresh parsley
2 egg yolks
sea salt and lemon pepper

Instructions
1. Fry bacon pieces to crispy and remove from pan leaving the drippings.
2. Saute' onion and garlic in same skillet. Remove from skillet and place with bacon.
3. Add chopped parsley and stir into bacon, onion and garlic. Set aside.
4. Rinse shrimp well and toss with splash of lemon juice not accounted for in ingredient list.
5. Combine egg yolks and 1 T. lemon juice. Whisking to combine. Set aside.
6. Place shrimp in hot skillet (medium to high heat) with bacon drippings and sauté until opaque. About 5-10 minutes or so. Remove from skillet.
7. Add butter, wine and lemon juice to skillet scrapping bottom for any possible renderings from bacon or shrimp.
8. Remove the skillet temporarily off the heat. Using a whisk, whisk in the egg yolk. Whisk quickly, add the yolk slowly.
9. Return the skillet to the heat and add back the shrimp, bacon, onion, parsley and garlic.

Stir around on simmer. Taste your sauce and add salt and lemon pepper to taste and take this opportunity to add more lemon juice if you feel it is needed.

This pairs quite well with other vegetables that traditionally are complimented by lemon such as asparagus, brussels sprouts, or fried broccoli: recipe 35

Comments:……………………………………………

……………………………………………………………………………………………

……………………………………………………………………………………………

……………………………………………………………………………………………

# Recipe 67: Smothered Pork Chops

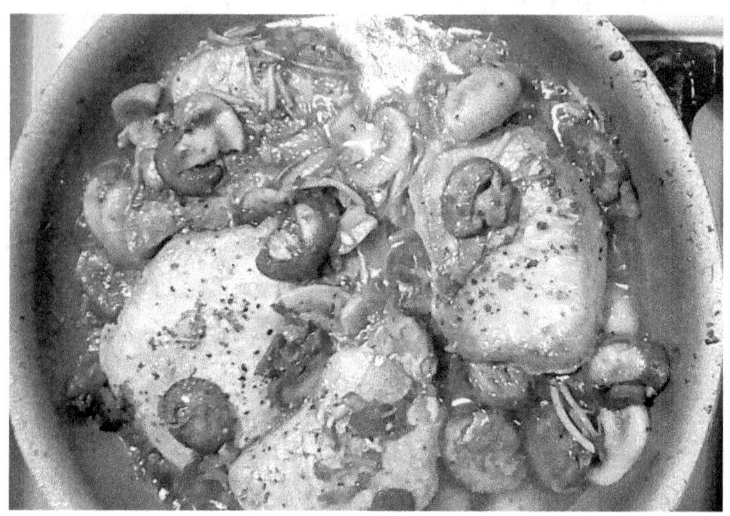

- 4 boneless pork chops
- 8 ounce package sliced mushrooms
- 6 T. oil
- Salt and pepper
- 1 garlic clove, minced
- 2 T. Real, Unsalted Butter
- ½ cup white wine or vermouth (could also substitute broth)
- 1 cup broth (I like to use chicken broth)
- ¼ cup chopped cilantro
- 1 t. lemon juice
- 1 T. cornstarch

1. Heat 3 T. oil in a hot skillet.
2. Salt and pepper your chops before adding to your hot skillet.
3. Brown the chops on each side. The first side about 7 minutes and the second side about 4.
4. Remove from skillet placing in a 350 degree oven for just 10 minutes. Remove to rest.

5.      While the chops are baking; toss sliced mushrooms, oil, garlic, salt and pepper in a bowl.
6.      After removing the chops from the skillet add the mushrooms.
7.      Allow the mushrooms to get a toasty brown.
8.      Sprinkle with cornstarch. Stir.
1.      Add the butter and the wine. Let simmer about 5-7 minutes. Stirring often.
2.      Toss in the cilantro and lemon juice.
3.      Cover chops with the mushroom gravy.

*This pairs well with Buttery Cabbage Recipe 12 or Mashed Cauliflower Recipe 47*

Comments:…………………………………………

……………………………………………………………………………………………

……………………………………………………………………………………………

……………………………………………………………………………………………

# Recipe 68: Spinach Salad

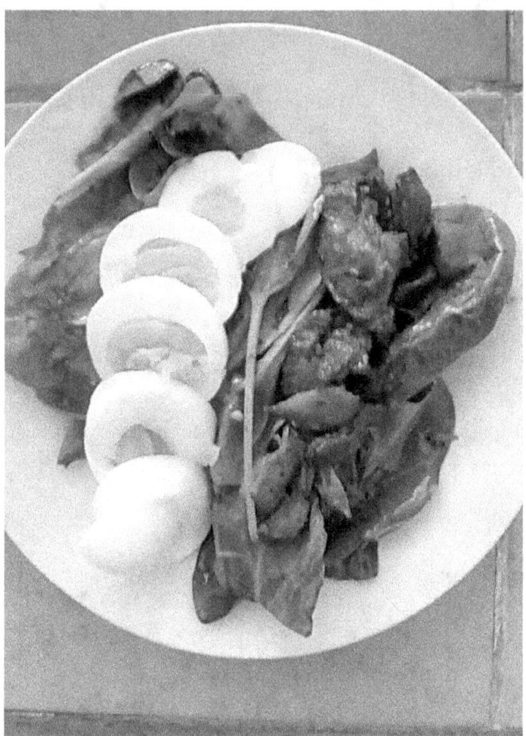

- 1 cup baby spinach
- 1 large egg, boiled
- 1 slice crispy bacon, crumbled
- 2 T. bacon fat drippings
- 1 T. red wine vinegar
- ¼ t. Dijon mustard
- Salt and pepper

If you only have 1 T. bacon fat add 1 T. oil.

- Combine bacon fat, vinegar, mustard, salt and pepper.
- Toss dressing with spinach. Arrange on plate and then top with sliced boiled egg and crispy crumbled bacon.

# Recipe 69: Stewed Yellow Squash

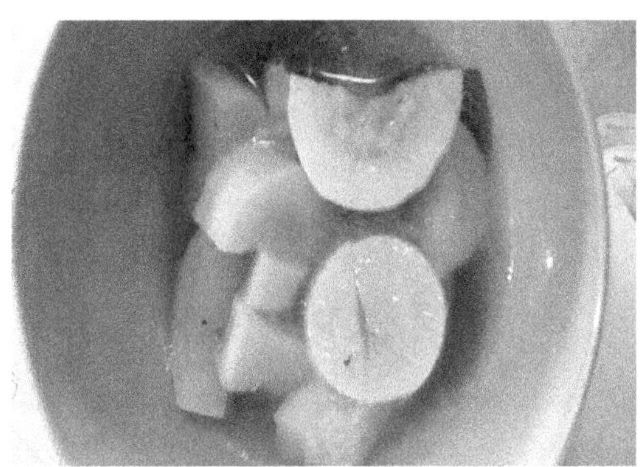

**INGREDIENTS**

- 1 cup Chicken Broth
- 1 medium Yellow squash
- 1 T. oil
- Salt, Pepper
- 1 large garlic clove
- 1 small bay leaf
- ¼ t. onion powder

1. Cut squash into bite size chunks. Place in sauce pan with enough chicken broth to cover. Squash should float. Add oil and seasonings.
2. Bring to a boil and then lower to a simmer. Simmer for about 25 minutes until the rind is quite tender.
3. Drain as much or as little of the broth as you wish but do remove the bay leaf and garlic clove.
4. Stewed squash pairs nicely with fish and seafood.

You can also add to your blender with half the broth made by stewing. Blend for a nice **Cream of Squash Soup**! Add more of the broth while blending to the consistency you like but it's best to start with half. You can always add broth but you cannot take it out! This is how I generally use any leftover stewed squash, or purposely make extra for soup.

# Recipe 70: Stuffed Mushrooms

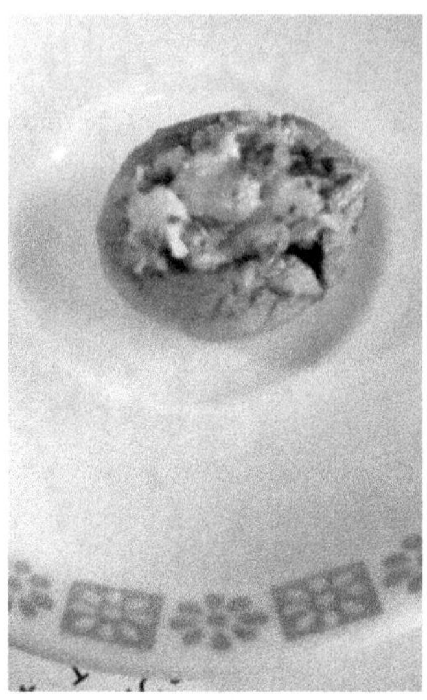

**INGREDIENTS for the mushroom caps:**

- Salt and pepper,
- 2 T oil
- 8 ounce package mushrooms; (whole. Your choice)


Comments:………….....……………………….....

………………………………………………………………………………………..

………………………………………………………………………………………..

………………………………………………………………………………………..

INSTRUCTIONS:

Remove the stems from your mushrooms and save.
Toss the mushrooms in a bowl with oil, garlic, salt and pepper
Spread onto a baking sheet. Set aside.

Preheat oven to 350 degrees. While the oven is preheating:

In the now empty bowl add:

**INGREDIENTS FOR THE STUFFING:**

- Mushroom stems
- 1 cup roughly chopped spinach or even romaine lettuce
- ¼ t. Onion powder
- ¼ t. garlic powder
- 1 t. Italian seasoning
- 1 T. apple cider vinegar

1. Put these ingredients into your chopper, blender, or food processor and do a rough chop so it is nearly pureed but definitely all minced together.
2. Using a butter knife stuff your mushrooms with this mixture, making sure to use the knife to push the mix down into the cavity of the mushroom.
3. Arrange the mushrooms onto your baking sheet.
4. Bake at 350 for 15 minutes.
5. Mushrooms should look golden brown and should be tender.

# Recipe 71: Swiss Chard with Balsamic

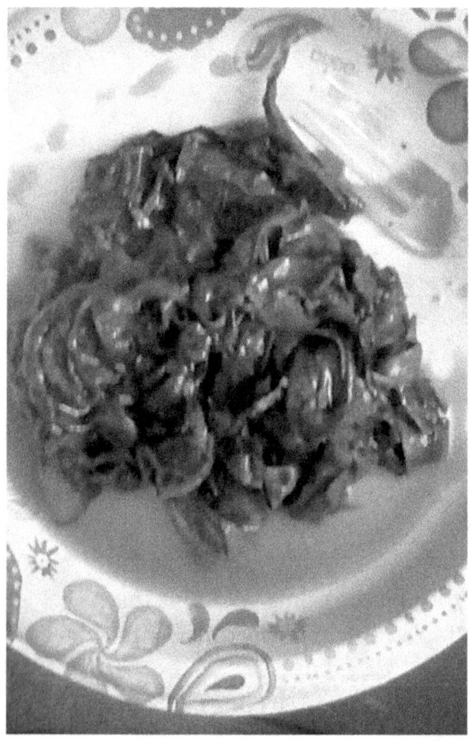

INGREDIENTS:

- 2 tablespoons olive oil
- ½ small onion, minced
- 3 fresh garlic cloves, minced
- 1 bunch swiss chard, stemmed and chopped well
- ½  cups chicken broth
- 2 tablespoons balsamic vinegar
- Salt and pepper

INSTRUCTIONS:

- Add oil, garlic, and onion to cold skillet. Heat to medium, stirring to coat.
- Add chicken broth to skillet. Heat to boiling.
- Evenly spread chopped Swiss chard over broth in skillet. Do not stir.
- Drizzle oil, salt and pepper to top of greens. Do not stir.
- Cover. Check every 5 minutes to see if chard looks appropriately wilted but do not stir. When greens are tender, remove from heat. Drizzle with Balsamic Vinegar, toss and serve.

Comments:…………………………………………

……………………………………………………………………………

……………………………………………………………………………

……………………………………………………………………………

# Recipe 72: Turkey Burger

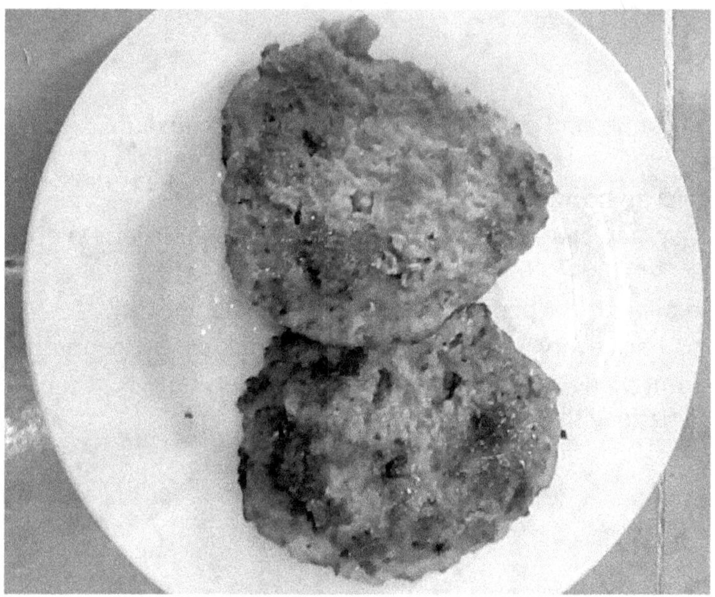

INGREDIENTS:

- ½ lb ground turkey (use the ground turkey found in the styrofoam tray, not the tube. Also use ground turkey that has never been frozen.)
- ¼ cup minced mushrooms (use a cremini or port mushroom for a deeper meaty flavor)
- Salt
- Pepper
- ½ t. Garlic powder
- ½ t. Onion powder

Mix all the ingredients and form about two patties.
Fry in a skillet in oil, or, use your grill.

The mushrooms not only add flavor but they also allow for a juicier burger.

Have you tried using lettuce as a bun? Summer is a great time for the lettuce bun. Light and refreshing. Not heavy. Layer a couple of outer leaves from your iceberg lettuce to make your bun!

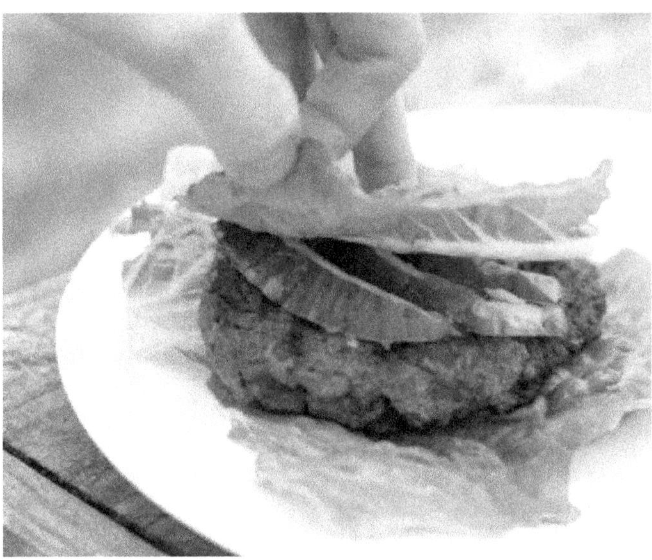

# Recipe 73: Turkey Chili

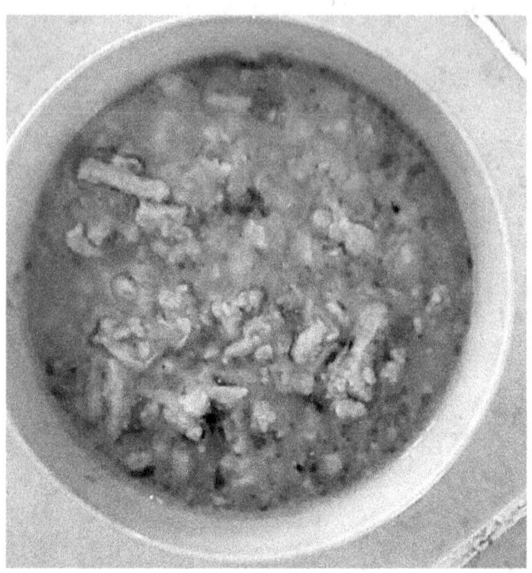

INGREDIENTS:

- 1 lb ground turkey (choose the ground turkey in the Styrofoam, not the tube)
- ¼ cup diced onion
- ¼ cup riced cauliflower
- ¼ cup diced celery
- ½ cup chopped cilantro
- 2 T. oil
- 2-3 T. cumin
- 1 t. garlic powder
- ½ t. ground ginger
- ¼ t. thyme
- 1 t. onion powder
- 20 ounces chicken broth
- 1 T. Apple Cider Vinegar
- 1 bay leaf
- ½ cup pureed carrots (pour a 15 ounce can of carrots with the liquid in your blender to puree or make from fresh cooked carrots using water)

**Instructions**

- Brown the ground turkey and onion in a skillet with the oil. Salt and pepper the ground turkey at this point (while it is cooking) along with the remaining seasonings.
- Once the ground turkey is browned, add the celery and cilantro.
- Add half of the chicken broth. If your preference is more broth (soup-ier) then go ahead and add more at this point. Remember that some of your broth will cook out.
- Add the vinegar, bay leaf and pureed carrots. Blend well.
- Add the cauliflower.
- Bring to light boil and let cook about 15 minutes. Cover and allow to simmer another 15-30 minutes.

Comments:…………………………………………

…………………………………………………………………………………………

…………………………………………………………………………………………

…………………………………………………………………………………………

# Recipe 74: Vegetable Beef Soup

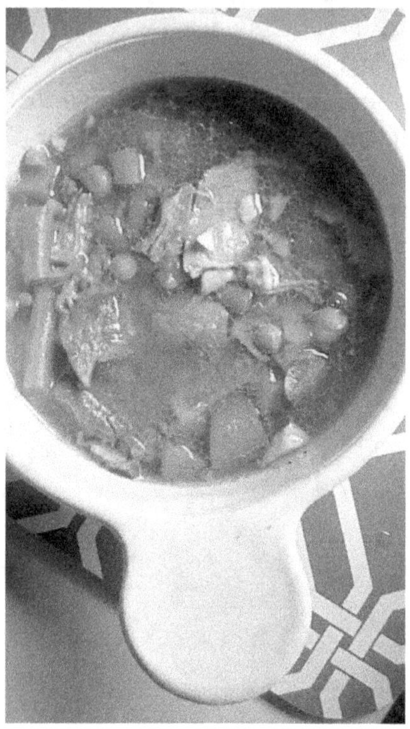

**INGREDIENTS**


1 or 2 Beef Shanks, bone-in
4 cups broth: Beef broth, chicken broth, vegetable broth or mushroom broth. I usually have plenty of chicken broth and find it works just fine.
1 (8-12oz) pkg of mushrooms, sliced
2 medium carrots, chopped
1 large onion, chopped
1 bay leaf
1 teaspoon thyme
Salt and pepper
1 T. oil

INSTRUCTIONS:

Place all of your ingredients in a crock pot and cook on low 6-8 hours, or on high 4-5 hours. Beef shank will just fall off the bone. If it doesn't, even though it appears done, it is because it has not cooked long enough. Turn the heat up and cook another hour or until tender and falling off the bone easily.

Comments:……………………………………………

………………………………………………………………………………………

………………………………………………………………………………………

………………………………………………………………………………………

# Recipe 75: Vegetable Hash

A chopper works nicely with all of the vegetables in this recipe! I don't recommend mixing the vegetables while chopping/dicing. Dice the mushrooms, remove. Dice the squash, remove. Etc…

- ½ cup diced yellow squash
- ½ cup diced zucchini
- ¼ cup diced cremini or portabella mushrooms
- 2 T. minced or diced onion
- Oil, salt and pepper

Toss all ingredients in a bowl.
Transfer to a hot skillet and sauté until tender. About 5 minutes.
I like to spread the vegetables in the skillet and press them into the bottom. Let it cook about 7 minutes on medium to high heat. This should cause a golden browning to the bottom. Then stir.

Add breakfast sausage and you have a nice breakfast with the leftovers.

**Comments:**...........................................

..............................................................................

..............................................................................

..............................................................................

# Recipe 76: Zucchini and Squash

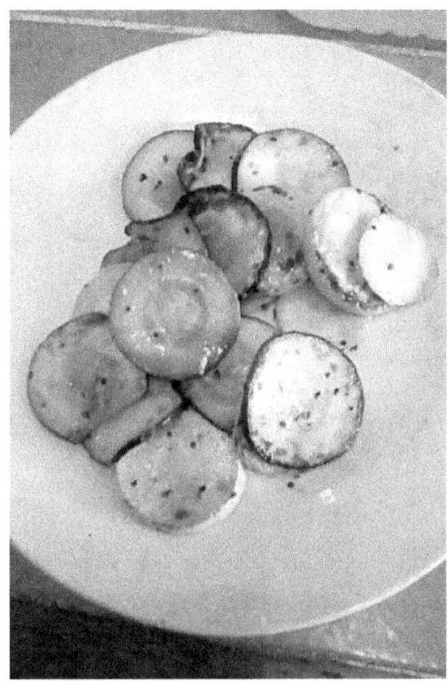

## INGREDIENTS

- 1 medium zucchini
- 1 medium yellow squash
- 4 T. oil
- Salt and pepper

Toss fresh zucchini and squash slices in oil, salt and pepper in a large bowl.
Heat a large skillet over medium to high heat and add the vegetables.
Spread the zucchini and squash out over the bottom of the skillet.
When vegetables start to brown, toss in the skillet and check for tenderness.
Should only take 5-7 minutes depending on how thin or thick you cut the squash and zucchini.

You can easily add ground turkey and seasonings but I highly suggest trying the basic recipe before you do that.

# Recipe 77: Zucchini Hummus

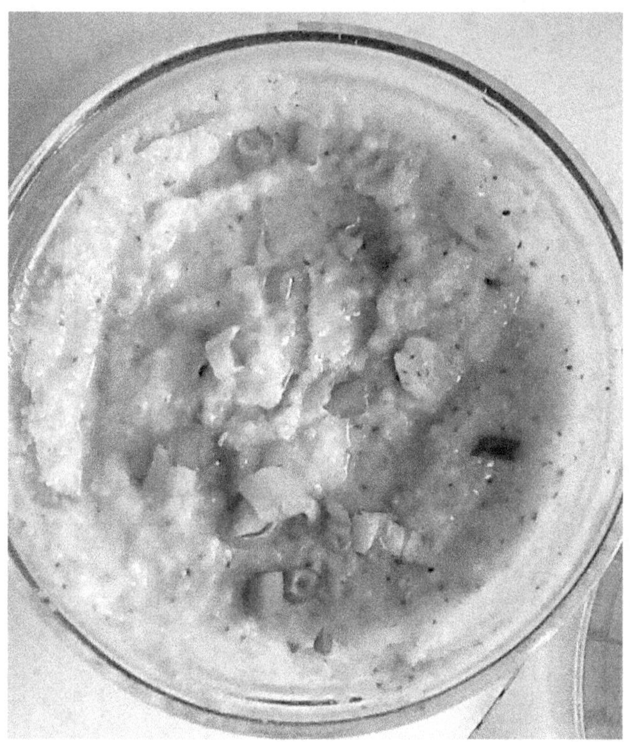

**INGREDIENTS**

½ small to medium zucchini
2 t. lemon juice
1 t. tahini or sesame oil
Pinch of salt
3 t. oil
¼ t. cumin
1 t. garlic powder

No need to cook the zucchini.

Place all ingredients in your blender until creamy smooth. Taste. Adjust seasonings, oil or juice to taste.

Especially good with radishes, romaine hearts, and scallions for dipping!

Comments:……………………………………………………

………………………………………………………………………………………

………………………………………………………………………………………

………………………………………………………………………………………

# Recipe 78: Zucchini Pancake

**INGREDIENTS**

- Cauliflower "Potato" Pancake recipe 13
- And add 1 cup shredded zucchini

Mix together and cook as you would a potato pancake.
A little oil in the skillet and cook to a golden brown on both sides.

Make this an entrée by adding ground turkey or ground pork.

Top with salad for a more hearty lunch or supper!

# SEEK AND FIND

| | | | | | | |
|---|---|---|---|---|---|---|
| N | I | E | T | O | R | P |
| H | E | F | I | B | E | R |
| E | F | R | E | V | C | A |
| A | R | E | C | E | I | T |
| L | E | I | A | G | P | H |
| T | S | N | R | E | E | Y |
| H | H | D | P | T | N | O |
| Y | M | E | P | A | E | D |
| S | O | S | K | B | R | R |
| I | C | S | C | L | G | S |
| O | V | C | A | E | Y | B |
| E | N | O | F | S | E | R |
| P | L | R | U | I | T | A |
| C | Y | P | P | A | H | C |
| H | J | N | B | O | D | Y |
| V | S | U | M | M | E | R |

| | | |
|---|---|---|
| 1. UNPROCESSED | 2. VEGETABLES | 3. HEALTHY |
| 4. PROTEIN | 5. RECIPE | 6. SUMMER |
| 7. ENERGY | 8. CARBS | 9. FIBER |
| 10. HAPPY | 11. FRESH | |

# Paula C. Henderson

Paula's books are available in kindle and paperback versions. You can see all of her titles on her author's page on Amazon:
**www.amazon.com/author/paulachenderson**

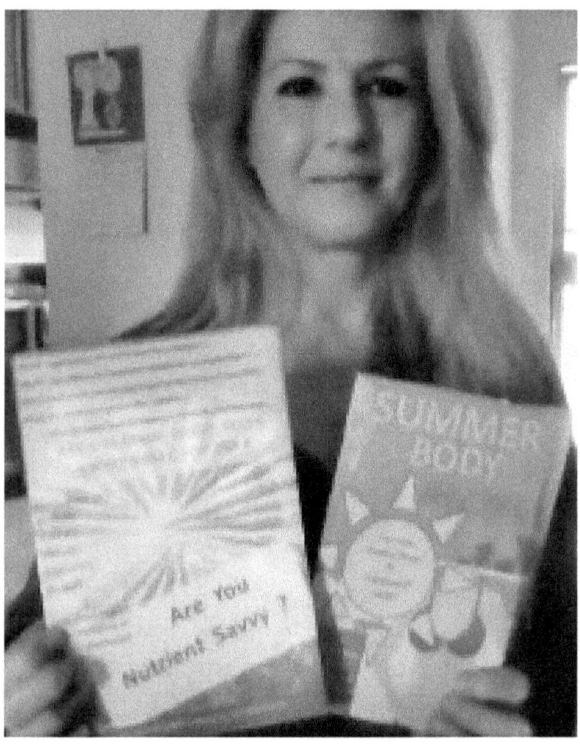

Paula C. Henderson makes her home in Las Vegas, Nevada.
Paula grew up in Illinois and then moved to Ohio where, as a single mother, raised her daughter.

Becoming a certified weight loss counselor started an interest in healthy food choices and a healthy lifestyle that continues today. Taking care of one's self is even more important when facing daily challenges. Through the years Paula has continued her education as a Nutritionist and health care advocate.

My first book was

"A Gluten and Dairy Free, Grain Free, Soy Free, and Nightshade Free *Grocery List*" available on Amazon in kindle ed:
 ISBN: 1542622727
https://amzn.to/2FKY8E1
And paperback ed: https://amzn.to/2rlRy2G

I followed that up with two cookbooks, **"Lettuce Amaze You"**
ISBN: 1540874931
https://amzn.to/2JTA5W3

and **"52 Low Carb Chicken Recipes"** https://amzn.to/2IdQvvj
ISBN: 1548330884

My most ambitious book and bestseller is **"Are You Nutrient Savvy?"**
ISBN: 1984004719
https://amzn.to/2rlgnLq

RECIPE NAME | PAGE # | MAKE AGAIN?

| RECIPE NAME | PAGE # | MAKE AGAIN? |
| --- | --- | --- |
| ......................................... | ............... | ..................... |
| ......................................... | ............... | ..................... |
| ......................................... | ............... | ..................... |
| ......................................... | ............... | ..................... |
| ......................................... | ............... | ..................... |
| ......................................... | ............... | ..................... |
| ......................................... | ............... | ..................... |
| ......................................... | ............... | ..................... |

MEAL PLANNERS, 4 WEEKS

*Week one*

# MONDAY

# TUESDAY

# WEDNESDAY

# THURSDAY

# FRIDAY

# SATURDAY

# SUNDAY

## *Week two*

# MONDAY

# TUESDAY

# WEDNESDAY

# THURSDAY

# FRIDAY

# SATURDAY

# SUNDAY

## *Week three*

MONDAY

TUESDAY

WEDNESDAY

# THURSDAY

# FRIDAY

# SATURDAY

# SUNDAY

# MONDAY

# TUESDAY

# WEDNESDAY

# THURSDAY

# FRIDAY

# SATURDAY

# SUNDAY

Paula C. Henderson

www.ingramcontent.com/pod-product-compliance
Lightning Source LLC
Chambersburg PA
CBHW051743250726
48659CB00001B/215